Advance Praise for
The Insider's Guide to Living Kidney Donation

"Inspirational, educational, and accessible. By combining personal stories with practical advice and clear information about the ins and outs of living kidney donation, this book proves to be an invaluable resource, answering questions you may never know you had about the process."

—ERIN WELSH, Ph.D.,
co-host of "This Podcast Will Kill You"

"Carol Offen and Betsy Crais have left no stone unturned in covering all facets of kidney donation and transplantation. Everything you need to know is right at your fingertips— a tool I wish existed 16 years ago when I donated."

—BRENDA E. CORTEZ,
author of *Howl the Owl*® series
and *Because of Organ Donation*

"This book is an absolute must for anyone touched by kidney disease. Along the lines of *Kitchen Confidential* by Anthony Bourdain, it is a joy to read, gives you practical knowledge and personal stories, and once you finish it you have a greater understanding of the beautiful world of transplantation."

—JOSHUA D. MEZRICH, M.D.,
author of *When Death Becomes Life:*
Notes of a Transplant Surgeon

"*The Insider's Guide to Living Kidney Donation* is a real gem, written by Carol Offen and Elizabeth Crais. From The Essentials to the future of living kidney donor transplant, this book covers the waterfront! A must read for anyone seeking a kidney transplant! Highly recommended!"

—**JAMES MYERS,** 2019 NKF Advocate of the Year;
American Association of Kidney Patients (AAKP)
Board of Directors

"As a nondirected kidney donor, I was thrilled to read *The Insider's Guide to Living Kidney Donation.* Donating a kidney is an experience like none other, but I wish I had had this guide when I donated. Whether you are a candidate for donation or simply curious, we finally have a source that answers every question I had prior to donating, and much more. Kudos to the authors!"

—**NED BROOKS,**
founder of National Kidney Donation Organization (NKDO)

"As a clinician and researcher focused on the care and outcomes of living donors, I am delighted that Carol Offen and Betsy Crais have created this clear, up-to-date, nontechnical guide to help potential donors understand key considerations as they approach the donation process. Guided by firsthand experiences of those who have been there, this resource will help donor candidates and families structure conversations with their transplant professionals."

—**KRISTA LENTINE, M.D., Ph.D.;**
St. Louis, Missouri

The Insider's Guide to

LIVING KIDNEY DONATION

The Insider's Guide to

LIVING KIDNEY DONATION

Everything You Need to Know If You Give (or Get) the Greatest Gift

CAROL OFFEN & ELIZABETH CRAIS

Foreword by Kenneth A. Andreoni, M.D., F.A.C.S.

*The content of this book is not intended to provide medical advice. Every effort has been
made to ensure the accuracy of the information, but this book is not meant to be a substitute
for consultation with a licensed practitioner. Please consult with your own physician or
healthcare specialist regarding the suggestions and recommendations made in this book.*

ISBN (Print): 978-1-09836-983-5

ISBN (eBook): 978-1-09836-984-2

BookBaby Publishing
First Edition 2021
Printed in the United States of America.

For further information about the authors' efforts in support of kidney donation,
please see www.kidneydonorhelp.com

For Paul, of course—and for Neil and Nora,
who have always been there for us.
—C.O.

To my mother, Barbara Schnell Crais, who passed PKD on
to my two sisters and myself, thereby inadvertently giving us a
PKD support group. She was a seeker of new information
and inspired us to continue that tradition.
—B.C.

Contents

Part Four: Community Connections

Part Five: Supporting Roles

Foreword

I HAD THE GREAT PLEASURE to be directly involved in the two fruitful transplant events that involved the authors of this book. I say "events" and not "surgeries" because the interactions we physicians routinely have with transplant recipients and their families are far more than the single transplant operation, as you will discover when you read about Carol and Betsy's own experiences. Their very real, and yet unique, journeys documented in this book, along with all the relatable information on donation and transplant that they have amassed here, clearly demonstrate why all involved in organ transplantation take this vocation so personally. As I tell my patients before their transplant, once they receive a transplant, they are married to a transplant center for the rest of that organ's functional life.

The relationship that all of us involved in organ transplantation develop is unlike that in any other field of medicine. Not only are long-lasting transplant physician and patient relationships the standard, but through organ donation events and even just day-to-day interactions, we develop connections with living donors, donor families, and the huge community of individuals who have had transplants themselves, and their family and friends.

When most people think of organ transplantation, they probably imagine state-of-the-art, cutting-edge technology involving delicate surgery and complex combinations of antirejection medications. This is true to a large extent; however, nothing in transplantation today is possible without the most personal of all selfless gifts that one person makes to another: organ donation. Whether this gift is between family members, lifelong friends, or individuals who will remain completely unknown to each other, one person is giving a part of his or her own being to another. This may sound over the top, but on the contrary, it is impossible to put into mere words the immensity of this gift, this "greatest gift." Kidney transplantation *doubles the life expectancy of the average adult with kidney failure* when compared to dialysis. *For children and younger adults, this advantage is more than threefold!* Kidney transplantation is a miraculous lifesaving event.

Carol and Betsy insightfully relate their stories of both living kidney donation and receiving a living-donor kidney transplantation. Their heart-warming journeys carefully incorporate accurate challenges as they traveled through their personal decisions to start the transplant process. They discuss the important education they received generally on kidney donation and transplantation and also the education that was personally directed at the concerns involved in their own events. Moreover, they have gathered a great deal of information that they learned both after their donation and transplant experiences and from others around the country, and make this vital information available to the reader. They bring us into the times around their operations, both as donor and as recipient, and share the very emotional and realistic physical challenges at that time. Even more importantly, Carol and Betsy discuss the challenges they experienced after leaving the hospital, a time when recipients and especially living donors can feel emotionally drained, even abandoned, after the surgical event.

The need for all donors is very real. Over 93,000 people were waiting for a kidney transplant in 2020, with another nearly 15,000 people waiting for another type of solid-organ transplant: liver, heart, pancreas, lung, or intestines. In 2019, 23,401 kidney transplants were performed, with almost 30% being from living donation. These 6,867 living kidney donations were the most in one year in the history of transplantation! The 16,534 deceased kidney donations were also the most ever. Unfortunately, more than 11,860 patients were removed from the waiting list without having a transplant. These patients either died while on the waiting list or became too ill to safely undergo a transplant. This eye-opening fact has been true for over fifteen years: just about as many people are removed from the waiting list as receive a transplant every year. If it were not for living donation, this number would strongly tip in favor of patients being removed without a transplant opportunity.

A person who is willing to be a living donor should clearly understand that removing a kidney is a real operation even though it may be minimally invasive laparoscopic surgery. The living-donor evaluation process may appear daunting to the donor candidate and even more so to the anxiously awaiting recipient candidate, but the thoroughness of that evaluation is mandatory for the health of the donor, optimal outcome of the recipient, and trust in the overall transplant system. Patients and families often do not want to hear the description of the operation, especially the possible complications, but without this truly informed consent, the integrity of the living-donor transplant process would not survive.

In the rare case that a living donor develops a kidney disease in the future, that donor receives priority if a transplant is needed. I remember one younger father who donated a kidney to his son, and over ten years later developed an unrelated autoimmune disease that caused his kidney function to decline. This type of illness would have given him the same problem if he still had both of his kidneys given that these diseases attack both kidneys simultaneously. Because the United Network for Organ Sharing (UNOS) waitlist system gives special priority for prior living donors, this donor was able to obtain a deceased-donor kidney without needing to start dialysis.

As I sit in the operating room lounge waiting to start a kidney transplant operation on a Veterans' Day, my gratitude is to the many who have served their country in the past, especially those who unfortunately paid the ultimate sacrifice, and also to the selfless deceased and living donors who allow others to live longer and with a higher quality of life. The information offered in *The Insider's Guide to Living Kidney Donation* can provide readers with the knowledge necessary to make this informed decision to be a donor—and to save a life. There are still heroes.

Kenneth A. Andreoni, MD, FACS
University of Florida, Gainesville
November 11, 2020

Preface

WE MET NEARLY TWO DECADES ago when our daughters were in the same Girl Scout troop (we bonded when we shared a pup tent during a camping trip). Some years later we learned that we also shared a passion for encouraging living organ donation that has resulted in this book.

How did we go from tent-mates to co-authors? Gradually. Very gradually. When Betsy faced declining kidney function in the early 2000s and had to consider dialysis and ultimately a transplant, the only books she found to inform her were renal-focused cookbooks or medical texts about kidney diseases, with short chapters about her condition (polycystic kidney disease, or PKD). There was little available on what to expect before and after dialysis or transplant, and certainly nothing that delved into topics related to emotions or family relationships.

Fortunately for Betsy, she at least could talk about her disease with her mother and two of her siblings, who also had PKD. Through them, she could at least get some of her personal questions answered. Later her sisters, one of whom had had a transplant, also came to help her when she had her surgeries. Having her siblings' care was a great blessing, and the best part was having them there to talk to, given that they had been dealing with PKD for years and could guide her expectations.

In contrast, when Carol faced the opposite situation a couple of years later—contemplating being a living donor for her twenty-five-year-old son, Paul—she knew no one who had donated a kidney. She had dozens of questions and could ask the professionals some of them but had no one to advise her who'd been through the experience. For Paul's questions, fortunately her family could call on Betsy, who talked to Paul to help allay his and his family's concerns. Most important, Betsy shared some encouraging examples of how her quality of life had improved after the transplant compared with her time on dialysis.

Not long after Betsy's transplant and recovery, she began thinking about her difficult experiences and the silver lining of having family members who could be her own invaluable support group. The awareness that most people, like Carol, do not have that critical support prompted us both to want to write a book that could help others know what to expect throughout the donation and transplantation processes. Both of us had been surprised and frustrated to find so little practical, nontechnical information and support in those pre-Google days.

Sure, a Google search now offers lots of information on living donation, but digging through the often-conflicting, frequently out-of-date, bewildering array of information is overwhelming. We wanted to do the vetting of that material and be able to offer readers clear, reliable resources.

Early on, Betsy drafted an outline and started thinking of people who might contribute various chapters, and Carol wrote an occasional op-ed piece on being a living donor. But because of day-to-day obligations, it would be several more years before Carol reached out to Betsy to talk concretely about an idea for this book. Neither of us knew that the other had already been thinking along the same lines.

Our ultimate goal in writing *The Insider's Guide to Living Kidney Donation* is to highlight the desperate need for living donors and to both encourage and support donation. Overwhelming statistics—like 100,000 people on years-long waitlists for a kidney and fewer than 25,000 transplants performed each year—become more understandable and meaningful when they are presented in terms of individuals' firsthand experiences. Besides providing authoritative information and sharing our own lessons learned, we decided to include other perspectives, with first-person accounts from people personally or professionally involved in the donation or transplant process.

From the beginning, we were on the same page in wanting to provide accessible and multifaceted information for both donors and recipients, because we were mindful that families, friends, and acquaintances of kidney patients are the best source of potential living donors. They are certainly the backbone of the patients' support system. In assisting donors, we reasoned, we would clearly be helping patients, too. We also wanted to reach readers who already planned to donate or to be a recipient as well as those just exploring the idea—and even some who may not have ever considered the possibility. We initially drew mostly on our own experiences in raising issues to be considered at all stages of a donation or transplant. In recent years, as we became immersed in the burgeoning kidney-support and living-donor communities, we were able to learn what "real-world" questions others were raising in workshops and online forums.

Within these parameters, we each had our own personal motivation and goals for the book. Betsy was particularly interested in addressing emotional and family issues—how a transplant might affect you personally and the impact it can have on your loved ones; Carol, a self-described wimp who feared the donor's medical evaluation phase as much as the surgery itself, wanted to provide details on tests and interviews to support and motivate others who might be similarly hesitant.

Although our experiences overlap, the reality is that potential living donors and transplant recipients have inherently different journeys. Living donation, by definition done by a healthy individual, is of course a choice; transplant, on the other hand, though technically a choice, is usually a critically needed and wished-for prospect for someone with kidney failure. Dialysis helps patients maintain some of their kidney function while awaiting transplant, but it cannot offer the same quality of life and long-term outcomes as a new kidney. The decision to seek a transplant and the steps in the process are determined by a patient's individual medical needs and circumstances. The medical issues naturally dominate, so frequently family and emotional considerations are given short shrift.

Because we fully recognize the implications of a decision to donate or have a transplant, we encourage everyone to consider the myriad factors that go into such a decision. We hope that having all the information contained in these pages will empower readers to be informed consumers, because information is power—never more so than in matters of health.

Working on this book has been a labor of love for roughly six years, as those day-to-day obligations occasionally pushed it to the backburner. In the beginning, we met every few weeks to talk generally about our vision for the book, gradually increasing the frequency and substance of our efforts. For the first four years nearly every meeting—with the notable exception of local TV news interviews conducted on Betsy's porch—was held at our second home and office, the since-closed Looking Glass Café, an inviting, community-minded coffee house in Carrboro, North Carolina. We moved on to the nearby Weaver Street Market co-op café for a while before having to retreat into self-quarantine when email, telephone, and Zoom formed our new meeting place.

Thanks for nurturing us for all those years, Looking Glass! We miss you and wish you were still around as we celebrate this book's publication.

Carol Offen and Elizabeth (Betsy) Crais
Chapel Hill, N.C.
December 2020

Part One:
The Essentials

CHAPTER 1

Why We Need More Living Donors

AN OHIO COUPLE TRANSFORM THEIR van into a cruising billboard, a woman in Pennsylvania posts her blood type on Facebook, a man offers thousands of dollars online…. These are just a few of the ways people try to find living kidney donors in this country.

Why resort to such unusual steps? The answer is simple. Today more than thirty million Americans have chronic kidney disease. Nearly 100,000 of them are on national waiting lists for a kidney from a deceased donor. About every ten minutes another person is added to the list. Meanwhile, nearly half a million people, many of whom may never be able to have a transplant, receive dialysis.

With fewer than 25,000 kidney transplants performed each year—from both deceased and living donors—most of the people on the list wait several years for a kidney: up to five to ten years in some states. That means that at least sixteen people in the United States die every single day simply because they did not receive a kidney in time.[1]

It doesn't have to be this way. Kidney transplants are hardly new—surgeons have been performing them for more than half a century. So why are they still helping only a fraction of those in need?

No Simple Answers

The principal reason for the long wait and the tragic deaths that result is obviously a shortage of available kidneys. But numerous factors account for that shortage. In the United States, only about 3 out of every 1,000 people die in a way that makes traditional organ donation possible—typically in a hospital following an accident—so the pool is very small. That is why we organ-donation advocates have long pushed for changes in our system of organ-donor registration. Rather than letting people opt out if they *don't* want their organs donated after their death, as is the policy in a growing list of countries, we have an *opt-in* system: you must select "yes" for organ donation when you apply for a driver's license or register online as a donor. In the United States 60% of people are now registered organ donors—even though 90% of adults in a national survey said they favor organ donation. In contrast, in Austria, for example, where organ donation is "presumed" unless someone opts out, about 99% of people are donors. It's not that simple, of course. An opt-out system is only as good as the built-in supports a government creates along with it,[2] so the change alone would not be a panacea but at least a start.

Persistent myths surrounding organ donation, such as the notion that life-saving measures might be withheld from a registered donor, surely compound the problem. Let's be clear: when someone is dying in a hospital, the doctors do not know or care whether that person is a registered organ donor. They have all sworn an oath to do no harm, so they will do everything they can to try to save the patient. If the person dies, the transplant team—a completely separate unit that has nothing to do with regular patient care—is not involved in organ donation until *after* the family gives consent. In fact, most deceased organ donors come from hospitals *without* transplant teams.

Whatever the reasons for the shortage, until the proportion of people who register as organ donors increases considerably or an artificial kidney becomes a reality, our best hope for reducing the tragic kidney shortage is through *living* donation. Because most of us are born with two kidneys, and we need only one functioning kidney, living kidney donation is the most common living organ transplant.

Dramatic strides have been made since the first one was performed in Boston in 1954, but we're always surprised that most people still don't know very much about living donation. This book's co-author, Carol, certainly didn't before her son's kidneys began to fail and she wanted to donate to him. And co-author Betsy didn't until she needed to find a kidney donor herself.

Advantages of Recipient Having a Living Donor

Most people don't realize that it's far better to get a kidney from a live donor than to have one from a deceased donor. With more live donors, not only could we ease the organ shortage, we'd see improvements in the recipients' recovery time and long-term prognoses. A live-donor kidney transplant has a greater chance of succeeding, partly because it has a better chance of working immediately. Also, because of the living donor kidney's usual quick start, the patient rarely needs to continue dialysis while waiting for the new kidney to be up and running, as is more often the case with a kidney from a deceased donor. As a result, both Betsy and Paul, Carol's son, like so many other live-donor kidney recipients, reported feeling better almost immediately after their transplant.

Perhaps best of all, a living kidney typically lasts much longer than one from a deceased donor: an *average* of fifteen to twenty years versus ten to fifteen years from a deceased donor. The jaw-dropping record is about fifty years for a living-donor kidney recipient. Deceased-donor kidneys rarely reach the thirty-year mark.

Having a living donor also usually offers the luxury of being able to carefully consider the date for the transplant surgery. It can be scheduled for the best time for both donor and recipient. If either of them is not well on the planned date, the surgery can be rescheduled for a few weeks later to ensure that the donor is in optimal health and the recipient is as strong as possible.

With a deceased-donor kidney, it's a game of chance as to when a patient will get "the call" that a compatible kidney is potentially available. Let's first explain what it means to be compatible, or to find an acceptable "match." Two different issues are involved: blood type and tissue type. The standard A, B, O, or AB blood types may be familiar from high school biology class, with type O being the universal donor. If you are a blood type O, like Carol, anyone can receive *your* kidney based just on blood type; if you are a type AB, you can *receive* anyone's kidney based on blood type. Unfortunately, if you are a type O, as Carol's son is, you usually can receive only from a type O donor. With few exceptions, a blood type A recipient can receive a kidney from an A or O donor, and a type B recipient from a B or O donor.

The second kind of compatibility for transplant is "tissue typing," known as HLA compatibility. It's the reason that a certain blood test, a "cross-match," is always required before a transplant can be performed, to ensure that the recipient doesn't have antibodies against that particular donor's organ. We'll talk more about that later when we get to chapter 3, "The Preliminaries." Some "highly sensitized" patients have higher levels of antibodies against nearly all other people, so finding a compatible donor for them can be extremely challenging.[3]

Once a patient gets the call, with no warning after being on the waiting list for years, he or she may need to hurriedly arrange for a possible one- to two-month leave from work and attend to family responsibilities such as child- or eldercare. Candidates usually need to be ready to go to the hospital the same day they are contacted, to allow time for testing, but of course not all kidney patients live near a transplant center. Although a kidney can safely be stored for twenty-four to thirty-six hours, the shorter the wait until it's transplanted in the recipient's body, the better: the lower the chance it may not function, the quicker it will usually "wake up" and function, and the better its chances for long-term survival. That window may allow ample time to put the kidney on a flight to anywhere in the country but woefully little time for candidates to deal with major obligations.

Even after getting the call, there is no assurance that the patient called will actually be able to have the transplant. Critical blood testing, including the cross-match, must be repeated. Because there are no guarantees, when a kidney offer is made at least one alternate patient is always called, too. Betsy has two sisters who, like her, have had kidney transplants. The first time that her sister Barbara got the call, she alerted her family and friends that the big day had arrived and then excitedly showed up at the hospital expecting to receive the kidney for which she'd waited years. Instead, after more testing and mounting anticipation she learned that another candidate ahead of her on the waiting list had had acceptable testing and would receive that kidney. She returned home distraught, and she resolved that whenever she got another call, she wouldn't inform family and friends until it was a sure thing. Some unfortunate kidney patients may repeat such a scenario seven or eight times before they get a kidney transplant.

Expanding Options

Almost every week brings news of advances that could make it possible for more people to find a compatible kidney and have a transplant. Thanks to technology, living kidney paired donation, in which unmatched donor-recipient pairs "swap" donors, has become common. And medical research is making it possible to increase use of certain deceased-donor organs that were once discarded. For example, in the last few years the option of transplanting a kidney infected with hepatitis C into someone without hepatitis C has become routine at many centers. Given that the disease can now be cured with few side effects, these kidney recipients are treated with drugs after their transplant surgery to cure (or prevent) the hepatitis, which usually takes just a few weeks of oral medications.

Of course, we still have a long way to go to narrow the gap between the 90% of Americans who reportedly favor organ donation and the much lower though rising percentage who actually register. Progress may have speeded up a bit because of Silicon Valley's help. For example, Apple's Health app makes it easy to register as a donor. Facebook, Twitter, and other social media platforms have also developed tools and public advocacy measures to make it easier to register as an organ donor, such as ORGANIZE's searchable registry of "social declarations" of desire to be a donor.

Major efforts are under way to bring more attention to kidney disease and the dire need for medical advances. The biggest development to date is the 2019 Executive Order on Advancing American Kidney Health. It includes the Public Awareness Initiative, a massive education effort to promote early detection and prevention, as well as a focus on medical innovation.[4]

The National Kidney Foundation's Big Ask, Big Give program and the Live Donor Champion workshops sponsored by several transplant centers for the past few years have focused attention specifically on helping kidney patients find a living donor. These free workshops train kidney patients' families and friends to use their personal contacts and social networks to spread the word about a specific patient's need for a kidney. Given that many individuals are uncomfortable with the idea of initiating this kind of conversation and using these methods for themselves, this strategy can be a remarkably effective approach.

Comparative Ease of Donor Surgery and Recovery

Regardless of the countless benefits for recipients, choosing to donate your spare kidney is still a major decision, and clearly not enough people are making it. One thing seems certain: If the families and friends of the more than ninety thousand kidney patients who were on the waiting list at the end of 2020 knew how comparatively easy and safe living donation has become in the past generation, the wait for a transplant would not be nearly as long. Thanks to major improvements in donor surgery and a robust donor-support network at most transplant centers, kidney donor hospital stays are now shorter and easier.

To be sure, it's not a walk in the park—major surgery never is—but with the minimally invasive laparoscopic technique used in nearly all cases, surgeons no longer need to remove one of the donor's ribs or make a large incision. That significantly reduces both the level of pain and how long it takes to bounce back. When Carol donated to her son in 2006, when she was fifty-eight, she was in the hospital for four days; now donor stay is typically one to two days. Incidentally, living kidney donors over fifty, like Carol, are increasingly common.

Follow-up after surgery has also improved substantially. After Carol was discharged from the hospital, a transplant nurse coordinator was available by phone 24/7, just as one is usually available for transplant recipients, so support and advice were just a phone call away. She had a post-op checkup at two weeks to make sure she was recovering smoothly and then at four weeks. At the four-week checkup, long since off the painkillers, she was given the green light to resume driving and a normal work schedule—and to follow up with her primary care provider as needed. Today donors typically have follow-up appointments with their nurse coordinator after two weeks and are then followed by the transplant center periodically for two years. The transplant community has made an active decision to follow living donors more closely with blood tests, blood pressure measurements, and quality-of-life questionnaires to provide increasingly safe care over time.

If Carol had needed to contact her nurse coordinator after that one-month check-up, however, she certainly could have. But by the next day after coming home, she was taking short walks and, had she not been the recipient's mother, she probably would have resumed her sedentary editor's job, at least on a reduced schedule, just two weeks later. In short, she had a comparatively easy post-op experience that was far better than she had anticipated.

Like most living kidney donors, Carol is still healthy and active several years after her donation. Living donors can help increase their recipient's life expectancy without reducing their own. Some studies have shown that donors live longer than their peers, probably because they must be in excellent health to be considered as a donor. Otherwise, there is no evidence of differences in lifespan between donors and comparable nondonors.

Nor do living donors need to compromise their quality of life. The most common constraints are to avoid extreme sports (not a problem for Carol) and NSAIDs (that's non-steroidal anti-inflammatory drugs, such as ibuprofen, because they are known to be hard on the kidneys). Carol has annual lab work to check her kidney function; a simple blood test measures her creatinine, which indicates the level of waste products in the blood and can be a sign of kidney problems. She doesn't take kidney medication or see a nephrologist (kidney medical specialist).

In other words, at seventy-two, she's healthy and has no medical concerns related to "missing" a kidney. In exchange, her son has had more than fourteen years, at this writing, living with her left kidney, which has given him a healthier, happier, productive life. So, yes, Carol would definitely do it again.

CHAPTER 2

Before You Make That Call

IF YOU'RE CONSIDERING DONATING YOUR kidney, before you start the process, let's examine some important questions:

What are the long-term health ramifications for the donor? Overall, there are few long-term issues. A donor's risk of developing high blood pressure and someday kidney failure is less than 1%,[5] even though that's higher than for similarly healthy people who haven't donated. Different ethnic groups have different rates of risk of kidney disease and its risk factors—for example, African Americans' rate of kidney disease is nearly four times that of white individuals—so it is very important for potential donors to discuss their individual risks in detail[6] with their provider and the transplant team.

Transplant centers say they lose track of two-thirds of donors after two years, which may mean that most donors feel no need to contact their centers, but more large, extended multicenter studies of donor risks are certainly needed.[7] The most common risk, as in many abdominal surgeries, is the development of a hernia in the incision that is made to remove the kidney, and a small risk of bowel injury or blockage.

In the extremely rare event that a kidney donor ever needs a transplant, he or she is given very high priority on the national waiting lists for a deceased-donor kidney, and also with the National Kidney Registry (for a live-donor kidney, if the donor participated in a paired donation through NKR). We say "extremely rare" because when one kidney is removed, the remaining kidney gets larger to take over some of the function of the removed one. Even though living donors lose some kidney function, the impact is usually not significant.[8]

Can you live a normal life with just one kidney? Of course, living with one kidney has minimal ramifications.[9] Of the thousands of people who are actually born with just one kidney, most enjoy healthy lives; in fact, before the widespread use of ultrasounds, it was not uncommon for such people to go through life without ever knowing they were short one kidney. Donors are encouraged to participate in most routine sports or physical activities (just not heavy contact sports to avoid injury). We know many kidney donors who run half-marathons and even marathons.

Can living donors go on to have a normal pregnancy? Absolutely. Centers now advise women to wait up to a year after the donor surgery before conceiving. Most women can then have a healthy pregnancy.[10] Many of Carol's living-donor Facebook friends have given birth after donation.

But of course, donating a kidney is not only a medical decision—it can also have emotional, social, and financial ramifications. So before you ever make a call to a transplant center—or even let your potential recipient know you're considering this step—carefully consider your reasons for donating, and think through what living donation might mean for you and your family, in both the immediate aftermath and the long term.

You know the general reasons for donating a kidney: the critical kidney shortage, the clear advantages of living donation versus a transplant from a deceased donor, the comparative ease of noninvasive donor surgery and recovery—and, as Carol can attest, the powerful gratification of helping someone live a fuller life. Donors of all types generally report a similar feeling and take tremendous pride in this special kind of personal accomplishment. In a long-term study of more than three thousand living kidney donors, most donors reported a "boost in self-esteem and an increased sense of well-being: 96% felt it was a positive experience."[11] This appears to hold true even when the recipient does not sustain a long period of post-transplant health and among the rare cases of donors who've experienced long-term health problems following their donation.[12] Regardless of the outcome, donors often describe the experience simply as "one of the best things I've ever done."

Individual reasons for donating vary widely, so it may be helpful to reflect on your own motivation. Maybe you want to do it for one of these common reasons:

- To enable your loved one to avoid a several-years-long wait for a kidney from a deceased donor.

- To come to the aid of a friend or acquaintance who has been on dialysis for a long time and has exhausted all other possibilities for finding a living donor.

- To do something "heroic" (note: most living donors would readily reject this term) by paying it forward and helping a stranger in need. If most organ donors might be considered altruistic, then nondirected donors—who may never meet their recipients—are surely the most altruistic of all.[13]

All good reasons—but whatever your own motivation, you should also consider any potential negatives. It may be helpful to list your individual pros and cons because there is no right or wrong here. As with any major decision, it is simply important to take your time and be sure you understand why you want to be a donor. This simple exercise may help you clarify your own reasons and separate the personal component from the immediate, overarching goal of finding a kidney for a particular recipient.[14] And it may help you focus on what information you need before you can make a decision.

No matter how strong your motivation, it is natural to have some trepidation and conflicted feelings. Briefly, here's how some would-be donors have resolved a few common concerns (we'll address these topics at length later in the book):

What if someone in my family needs a kidney someday?

Some donors, particularly those whose family members are at risk for kidney failure, have participated in a voucher program operated by the National Kidney Registry, or NKR, and certain transplant centers. In this case, you could donate an organ before the need arises, and the system would give you "credit" for your loved one to receive a matching kidney if and when the need arose. That person could receive priority a few months, years, or even decades later. Although there is no guarantee that a match will be available precisely when needed, the voucher system definitely offers a significant advantage. For donors who do not have kidney disease in their family, many say that a vague "what if" down the road should not prevent them from doing a generous act for someone in need *now*. They feel confident that should a need arise in their own family someday, another selfless individual will come forward just as they are doing now.

I don't know if I can afford the lost pay and additional expenses.

Most donors research the growing options for financial assistance for any lost pay and for significant incidentals, such as childcare, or travel expenses if they live far from the transplant center. Expanded financial help is available through the National Living Donor Assistance Center (NLDAC) and a host of other sources. For donors who use paired donation, NKR, for example, provides extensive protections. Some donors also raise money through GoFundMe campaigns.

My recipient might put the new kidney at risk by neglecting his or her health.

Realistically, there are many unknowns, often unrelated to the recipient's lifestyle, that might cause a kidney to be rejected. Studies have shown that the vast majority of living donors have no regrets no matter the outcome. We know a donor who was afraid that her brother with diabetes would be careless about his post-transplant health, but she decided she was comfortable with her decision to donate regardless of what happened after the transplant. Interestingly, he turned out to be a very responsible caretaker for her kidney.

Once you've carefully examined your reasons to donate, if you haven't yet discussed the idea with your partner or family members, now is the time. Knowing the basics about donation should help you answer some of their questions and perhaps reduce their concerns. If your recipient is not an immediate family member, your spouse may initially be uncomfortable with the idea—especially if you're considering being a nondirected donor, which may be more difficult for your loved ones to understand and accept. One would-be donor said that having her reluctant husband participate in her meeting with the surgeon helped reassure him. Together you can decide when to involve your children or other family members in these discussions.

If possible, talking to someone who has donated a kidney could be extremely helpful for you and your partner both now and later in the process. A previous donor might raise some issues, both positive and negative, that you haven't considered yet. Carol has often wished she had had that option. That's why we both volunteer as mentors to potential donors and recipients. Ultimately, the decision of whether to donate is an individual one that can be made with as little or as much input from others as you choose. Remember, *you* know your reasons best.

CHAPTER 3

The Preliminaries

KNOWING THE TYPICAL STEPS IN the donor evaluation/preparation may also help you make your decision. This is usually a months-long process, and it's wise to take one step at a time, but don't hesitate to start the process for fear that there's no turning back. When Carol was considering donating her kidney to her son, the reassuring knowledge that she could always change her mind up until she made the donation—an assertion repeated by several of her providers—gave her the self-confidence to proceed with her decision to donate. In the two years after her son's kidneys failed, Carol passed through several stages in her decision to donate (strong resolve–some hesitation–weak conviction–strong resolve), which seemed to fluctuate by the day. Eventually, she found that she had passed almost imperceptibly from wavering to a strong conviction that she wanted fervently to donate to her son.

One of the first pieces of information to determine is where the transplant will take place. If you already know, check out the transplant center's website. Also, the United Network for Organ Sharing (UNOS) has a very clear, thorough website with valuable information for both living donors and recipients. If something is unclear or problematic, you can raise a question about it when you contact the transplant center.

Now that you have taken the essential mental and emotional steps, and you are relatively sure of your intentions, you're ready for the preliminary stages of finding out if you can be a living kidney donor.

The Initial Contact

If the transplant center is nearby, consider not yet telling your potential recipient and his or her family of your desire to be evaluated. As Betsy knows from experience, raising a patient's hopes prematurely can backfire should plans to donate fall through. If you are considering being a nondirected donor, it's usually preferable to contact the closest center, because you will probably need to do much of the testing there and will be required to remain nearby for about a week after the donation. If you have the resources and the flexibility to travel and want to identify the "best" transplant center in your region, you could consider general reputation, such as *US News & World Report*'s annual hospital rankings, or anecdotal reports from previous donors through online support groups. Also, ask the transplant center how many kidney transplants it does in a year; you can find detailed information online on the volume of living-donor and deceased-donor transplants[15] performed at U.S. centers.

When you explore the transplant center's website, search for the section on Living Kidney Donation and read all of it. It will include a note about either calling the center or clicking a link for more information. Many if not most centers now provide an online registration form with a detailed health and family history questionnaire. If you're not ready for that step, look for an option to just make initial contact with someone from the transplant team.

Your first personal encounter with the transplant team could be a brief and fairly casual telephone conversation with the transplant donor coordinator. A registered nurse, the donor coordinator is the transplant team member a living donor interacts with most. (In a later chapter, we'll tell you all about the rest of the team, whom you'll meet later.) The donor coordinator talks to potential donors every day and should be happy to answer your questions. You'll probably be asked to whom you want to donate, whether you are related to the recipient, and where you live. To find out if living donation is even feasible for you, if the center doesn't use a preliminary online questionnaire, the donor coordinator will do a brief initial screening with a few questions you can answer over the phone. Some medical conditions will automatically eliminate you from consideration as a donor—for example, diabetes, severe hypertension, certain cancers, heart disease. Similarly, donors usually must be at least eighteen years old and under sixty-five, although some centers will consider potential donors well into their seventies and others may prefer that young donors be over twenty-five. If you pass the initial screening, the donor coordinator will send you a link or an information packet that will address many of your questions.

During this early period, it can be frustrating and disappointing if you don't get a call back from a coordinator as soon as you'd expect. Transplant coordinators often have hundreds of people awaiting evaluation. There may be another reason, too. Coordinators need to walk a fine line between being accessible and helpful but not seeming to encourage—and surely not pressure—the potential donor. They want to be sure that the impetus comes from the potential donor, who should be the one driving the process at this point.

The Health Questionnaire

Assuming that no red flags have surfaced during the phone screening or as you reviewed the information packet, you are ready for the health questionnaire. It covers your own and your family history but is more detailed than forms required when you start at a new medical practice. It can be completed online or printed and mailed. If completing the form online, be prepared with information such as surgery dates and family members' diseases just in case the form needs to be completed in one session.

Unlike the absolutes in the initial screening, certain types of medical history on the health questionnaire are less clear-cut and their risks more subjective. Conditions that are acceptable at one transplant center may not pass muster at another—for example, a single past kidney stone (which ruled out Carol's husband as their son's donor); melanoma (this eliminated Betsy's husband as her donor); controlled hypertension; heart disease, which covers a range of conditions; and certain mental illnesses.

The donor coordinator will handle the next steps in the donor evaluation process. Depending on the transplant center and the donor's schedule, the testing and interviews may take place over a couple of days or, more commonly, several weeks or even a few months, as Carol's did. Some centers permit a potential donor to have the tests done on two consecutive days, particularly if they are coming from out of town. If you do live far from the recipient, be sure to clarify certain logistical aspects early on—such as which tests can be done locally instead of at the transplant center, or how long you would need to stay nearby after the surgery. Given that travel and lodging costs can quickly add up and are not covered by most health insurance plans, having that information sooner rather than later can help you make a decision on whether to donate, when to schedule the surgery, and whether to line up financial assistance.

Lab Work to Test Compatibility with the Recipient

If your medical and family history are acceptable, the donor coordinator will order initial lab work to verify that your blood and tissue type are compatible with your intended recipient's, plus a cross-match to make it less likely that the recipient's body would reject your kidney.

As we mentioned, compatibility matching entails more than knowing your blood type, though that's the first step. Three main tests are required:

Blood typing (ABO). A simple blood test can confirm whether you have type A, B, AB, or O (incidentally, Rh factor—that is, negative/positive—doesn't matter here).

Tissue typing (HLA, or human leukocyte antigen). HLA antigens are proteins on most cells in the body, such as white blood cells, the lining of blood vessels, and the cells inside organs. Six of these one hundred HLA antigens were historically determined to be the most likely to cause rejection, so these are the main ones tested to determine the degree of matching, but most transplant centers now test for additional HLA antigens to use for detailed antibody considerations.

Cross-matching. In this critical step, the patient's blood is mixed with that of the identified potential donor to see if the recipient's antibodies will attack the donor's white blood cells. You don't want a positive reaction because that would signal an increased risk of early rejection.

If you are cleared to proceed, the donor coordinator will move full steam ahead now. Have you found a living kidney donor to talk with yet? If not, the donor coordinator may be able to arrange for you to speak with one. Alternatively, the National Kidney Foundation (NKF) has a nationwide program of volunteer donor mentors, NKF Peers (call 855-NKF-PEER), who can easily arrange a confidential, free telephone consultation. Many smaller, local organizations, such as the Donate Life/WELD (Women Encouraging Living Donation) chapter in which Carol is active, offer the same service.

Congratulations on completing these all-important first steps!

CHAPTER 4

What If You're Not a Match?

OF COURSE, EVEN WITH THE best of intentions, not everyone who makes it this far in the evaluation process can donate. Some reasons are more of a deal-breaker than others and, happily, new options are coming about all the time. Of all the roadblocks to someone becoming a donor, the first one that many people think of is "matching." But how much does matching matter anymore?

What Does It Mean to Be a Match?

When we say someone is a "match," as we explained, we could be referring to one of two kinds: blood type or tissue typing. Blood testing is relatively simple and just takes a professional to draw blood and determine the type. The universal donor—type O—can give to any blood type, but with rare exceptions, type A can only give to A or AB; type B to B or AB; and so on. That generally means that a type O recipient, like Carol's son, could receive only from a type O donor, like Carol.

Once the blood-type hurdle is cleared, tissue typing comes into play. Instead of the alphabet soup of blood types, tissue typing is all about numbers: the number of certain antigens (proteins on the cells), out of 6, that are a potential match. Getting all 6 is rare in deceased donation. Because we inherit 3 of these 6 antigens from each of our parents, biological siblings naturally have the best chance of getting a 6-antigen match, the so-called "perfect match." (A true perfect match exists only in identical twins. In any other case, these patients could reject their new kidney if they don't take antirejection medications.) Siblings who are not identical twins have

- a 1 in 4 chance of a 6-out-of-6 match
- a 2 in 4 chance of matching 3 of 6 antigens, and
- a 1 in 4 chance of not matching at all.

The higher the number out of 6, the better the match, especially for early success. This traditional gold standard exists because of the body's instinct to destroy foreign substances. That's why nearly all transplant recipients necessarily follow a lifelong regimen of antirejection medications to purposely suppress their immune response, so their body will not reject their new kidney, be it from a deceased donor or a living one.

That gold standard is becoming less critical. There's currently no magic number—it's not uncommon now for transplants to be done with *no* matching antigens, although well-matched living-donor kidneys still have less chance of rejection and the best chance for surviving the longest.

The third—and critical—condition for receiving any kidney is cross-matching, the important blood test we mentioned earlier that must be repeated before a transplant. The recipient's and the donor's blood are mixed, and—yes, it seems counterintuitive—we want a *negative* crossmatch. A positive cross-match would mean that the patient's antibodies are attacking the cells of the donor, so naturally a transplant with that kidney would *not* be recommended. Technically, cross-matching is not always clearly positive or negative but can often be a "low positive" result. Your transplant physicians will look very closely at which antibodies against this particular donor you have—that is, "donor-specific antibodies"—and will talk to you about how serious they consider this result.

Before improvements in antirejection medications, the vast majority of successful living donor transplants, not surprisingly, came from blood relatives. That's still the largest group, but increasingly spouses, in-laws, friends, neighbors, colleagues, and nondirected donors (formerly known as "altruistic")—that is, Good Samaritans who donate to an unknown recipient—are becoming living donors.

Could a Kidney Exchange Be the Answer?

In addition to the advances in medications, modern computer software has taken the living transplantation field one giant step further, opening up new possibilities for donating a kidney. Not that long ago, if a potential donor wasn't a match for an intended recipient for whatever reason, the kidney patient was out of luck and might need to stay on dialysis. End of story. But then kidney paired donation came along early in the new millennium with a few dramatic but limited efforts. These "kidney swaps," or exchanges, allow a kidney patient whose potential donor is healthy, but not a good match, to receive a kidney from a compatible living donor who, similarly, is not a match for his or her intended recipient. In other words, let's say you want to donate a kidney to your friend Alice, but you're not a match. However, you know that Bob is a match. Bob may be willing to donate to Alice if you donate to his friend John. If you're a match for John, that's simple—problem solved.

If, however, that second hopeful pairing isn't a match, what if you could involve more people? That's where computers come in. Complex algorithms are now able to look at the myriad matches possible among all the potential donors and recipients—at one hospital or at other hospitals participating in the matching program. Typically, one nondirected donor initiates the paired exchange or even a domino donor chain involving still more people.

That means now more and more people can be living kidney donors. The increasingly long donor chains in recent years are the logical extension of early paired donation. The record for the longest verified kidney transplant chain in the United States was set in 2015, by the National Kidney Registry: 35 living-donor transplants.

Most of us can fathom a kidney donor's motivation in paired donation, but when it comes to nondirected donors, many people are incredulous that they would give so much to someone they don't know, with seemingly nothing in return. Most nondirected donors will tell you that that's hardly the case. The majority of these donors report that they experience that same powerful feeling of gratification that Carol and other directed donors share.

CHAPTER 5

Tackling Potential Donor Obstacles

Are You Healthy Enough to Donate?

ONCE INITIAL TESTS CONFIRM THAT living donors are a match for their recipient or a paired donation, they still have to pass numerous medical and psychological tests to ensure that they are healthy enough to be a donor—both for their own sake and that of the recipient. Unfortunately, not all potential living kidney donors are healthy enough to donate. Jenine Lewis's kidney function was found to be too low—*the night before the surgery*—to donate to her friend (Jenine tells her story in Part Five). Although she was crushed when the surgery was abruptly cancelled, she later was grateful for the transplant team's clear commitment to protecting her health. It's not uncommon for donor candidates to learn about a health problem in the course of the evaluation. That discovery may save their lives by prompting them to get early treatment for their diabetes or hypertension, for example. Jenine's experience prompted her to commit to taking better care of her kidneys.

Heart, kidney (even kidney stones), and liver disease, and some cancers and chronic infections, generally preclude people from being living organ donors. And certain health conditions that typically disqualify someone from being a kidney donor—such as diabetes and hypertension—have been on the rise in the United States. Obesity, another increasingly common condition, does not necessarily rule someone out as a kidney donor, because many transplant centers will work with potential donors to help them lose weight and improve nutrition. We know of many donors who've managed to lose more than thirty pounds to be able to donate safely. Nevertheless, the U.S. public health crisis stemming from some of these conditions has surely contributed to the low numbers of living donors.

Partly because these risk factors are often more prevalent in minority groups, minority individuals experience higher rates of kidney failure, which necessarily also leads to low numbers of minority donors. For example, African Americans, who are nearly four times as likely as whites to develop kidney failure,[16] represent 13% of the U.S. population but 35% of the people on dialysis due to kidney failure; they are twice as likely as whites to be diagnosed with diabetes. Similarly, about 17% of Hispanic Americans have diabetes, and their risk of developing kidney failure is 1.3 times that of non-Hispanics.[17] As a result, African Americans, Hispanics, Asians, Native Hawaiians, and Other Pacific Islanders together represent more than half of those on the kidney transplant waiting list.

We have a vicious circle as the very factors that make minorities more likely to suffer from kidney failure obviously eliminate many potential donors. The common misconceptions and various other issues mentioned earlier combine to dissuade still others. For example, in 2019 41% of whites had a living donor transplant compared with 14% of African Americans.

Clearing Financial Hurdles

Most people believe that no one should make money from donating a kidney to save a life—it's actually illegal in most countries—but neither should anyone *lose* money. It should be financially neutral. Yes, the recipient's health insurance (including Medicare and Medicaid) normally pays for the donor's testing and surgery costs, but usually not additional expenses. Some insurance companies have started reimbursing lodging and travel expenses for a covered recipient's kidney donor who lives far away, sometimes even the expenses of a companion. It's always worth checking with insurers.

More broadly, the National Living Donor Assistance Center, NLDAC, has long provided federal grants for travel and lodging of eligible potential donors. That's certainly been a big help, but travel costs affect only a small portion of donors. NLDAC recently acceded to advocates' demands for expanding its financial assistance and in late 2020 began covering lost wages and certain related expenses, like childcare; it's also expanded eligibility. The National

Kidney Registry first began covering lost wages and related childcare and eldercare in 2019. Reimbursing living donors for missed pay if they don't have paid sick leave or short-term disability insurance can be a game changer for a lot of people.[18]

Donation advocates continue to lobby for significant and widespread government reimbursement of related expenses[19] so that no one need ever mount a GoFundMe campaign to make donation possible. In the meantime, new organizations have emerged to provide meaningful assistance with assorted costs, in a growing effort to surmount financial obstacles to living donation. Typically, states vary markedly in their policies on paid leave and tax deductions and credits.

Federal employees are allowed up to thirty days of paid leave for organ donation, and many states have slowly followed suit. More than half of states offer one to six weeks of paid donor leave for their state employees; most grant up to thirty days. *Private* employers are another question, however. Only a few states require private employers to provide paid leave for organ donors, or even offer incentives to encourage it, so there is still much work to be done.

Most state tax codes at least make expenses related to organ donation tax deductible, but that's hardly sufficient. For starters, we'd like to see tax *credits* for donors.

Cash payments to organ donors will probably always be illegal in the United States because of the uncomfortable idea of paying for body parts[20] and the inevitable differential between those who can and cannot afford to pay. But in addition to expense reimbursement and tax credits, what about scholarships, extended health coverage—and any other reasonable alternatives?

If the risk of additional expenses could derail your plans to donate, learn what your options are. And be sure to raise your concerns with the transplant team.

CHAPTER 6

Who's on the Transplant Team?

NOW THAT YOU'VE CLEARED THE preliminary hurdles in becoming a kidney donor and are ready for the in-depth evaluation, you'll soon meet the rest of the transplant team. Before you have the interviews and appointments, it will be helpful to learn a little about each professional so you'll have a better idea of *whom* to ask *what*. At any given kidney transplant center, by the way, we say *the* transplant team when we refer to the group of transplant professionals who share their expertise with the goal of ensuring a successful transplant while safeguarding the donor's health. In reality, many centers actually have *two* transplant teams associated with each kidney transplant: one for the recipient and the other for that person's donor. It is paramount that a potential donor not feel pressured into donating an organ, and having a separate roster of professionals helps to ensure that.

Below are brief descriptions of the key transplant team members whom potential donors will probably meet over the course of a donor evaluation and surgery. After each description, we've suggested a few questions you may want to ask as a starting point. Depending on your situation, you may find that some questions are equally or more appropriate for another member of the team; feel free to pose the same question to more than one person.

Transplant nurse coordinator. By now you've met the team's gatekeeper, the registered nurse who works with potential donors (*the donor coordinator*). This is your go-to person for answers to medical and logistical questions, advice, and referrals to other members of the team. You may work with the same donor coordinator throughout the evaluation and even two years beyond the transplant. He or she will examine you, order tests, help prepare you, and explain the results and any ramifications.

Potential Questions: Can I have some of the tests done at my local hospital if I live far from the transplant center? What happens if I change my mind about donating? Could I talk to someone who's donated a kidney?

Ask anything and everything. If the donor coordinator doesn't know the answer, he or she will either find out or refer you to the appropriate member of the team.

Independent living donor advocate (ILDA). The ILDA role was created in 2007 to ensure the protection of living donors and prospective donors. Unlike the donor coordinator, the ILDA is not a nurse, so is not involved in the medical and logistical aspects of the process. The role resembles that of a social worker, and in practice most ILDAs wear more than one hat, frequently doubling as the donor social worker. Only very large transplant centers have a person who serves solely as the ILDA.

Much like the donor coordinator or the donor social worker, this person is there to represent the donor's best interests, to advocate for your interests. The ILDA is also responsible for ensuring informed consent by making sure that you have been given complete information, fully understand it, and have thought through your decision to donate. Your discussions are confidential. If the ILDA identifies reasons that you should not donate, he or she will make that known to both you and the transplant team.

Because the position was created after both Carol's donation and Betsy's donor's, neither of us personally dealt with an ILDA during our donations. Long before the ILDA role was created, however, many transplant centers recognized the importance of avoiding conflicts of interest by assigning different professionals to work with the donor.

Potential Questions: What happens if someone else is considering donating? (Many centers will evaluate just one person at a time.) What happens if I develop kidney disease down the road and later need a transplant? What if I'm turned down—can I appeal?

———————————————

Donor social worker. The donor social worker's many responsibilities encompass both practical and social needs. He or she can help you learn your options on logistical issues that may arise during the testing and post transplant, such as transportation to and from the transplant center, caregiving, or childcare. Logistical issues are often an additional source of stress at a difficult time, particularly if the recipient is a family member, as in Carol's case. In general, the social worker can let you know your options and what programs are available to you, including disability programs, government funding for various services, and financial assistance for lost wages or child-care expenses. For program details and applications, however, you will probably work with the financial coordinator.

Potential Questions: If I am donating to my spouse, will we need to have a caregiver after we get home? I'll need childcare after surgery—what should I do? Will I have more trouble getting health insurance or life insurance because of being a donor?

———————————————

Nephrologist. Nephrology is the study of the kidneys; a *transplant* nephrologist specializes in the unique issues of kidney transplantation, a rapidly evolving field of study. As with the other transplant team members, you will usually be assigned a separate transplant nephrologist from that of the recipient and will meet with him or her to discuss your surgery; in smaller transplant programs, you may instead have a general nephrologist who is familiar with kidney donation.

Potential Questions: What impact will the kidney removal have on my kidney function? Will I have lifelong dietary restrictions? Will I need to be seen regularly by a nephrologist?

Transplant or living donor surgeon. This is the surgeon who will perform the donor nephrectomy (kidney removal), examine you, and explain the procedure and its risks. Your surgeon will also decide what additional tests, if any, you should have before the team makes a final decision. After the surgery you will be followed by the transplant team.

Potential Questions: How is the surgery done? How long will I be on pain meds? How many living-donor nephrectomies have you performed?

Donor psychologist or psychiatrist. Because it is critical that a potential donor have the mental and emotional capacity to make this important decision, a psychological evaluation is an essential part of the overall evaluation. A psychologist or psychiatrist will assess your mental and emotional health and affirm that you are capable of making and understanding the decision. This professional may also be available for consultation throughout the process.

Potential Questions: Do you share my comments with the rest of the team? How can I reach you if I have a concern? How can I reassure my spouse about my decision?

Transplant financial coordinator. The financial coordinator will explain how the administrative process works, the costs involved, who is responsible for what, and what additional costs you might encounter. He or she will probably inform you that you should not receive a bill from the hospital for either the testing or the surgery. If one does arrive in error, you will be told where to forward it. The bottom line is that the recipient's health insurance—whether private, Medicare, or Medicaid—usually covers the donor's evaluation (which alone can run as high as $15,000 per potential donor), the surgery, and post-op costs.

If you live near the transplant center, have employer-provided paid leave, and have no additional child care expenses, you will probably have no additional expenses. If that is not the case, be sure to talk with the financial coordinator about sources of financial assistance.

Potential Questions: How can I get financial assistance for while I'm not working? If the evaluation discovers a possible medical problem that needs to be treated, who pays for additional tests? If I later need additional surgery related to my donation, for how long will it be covered by my recipient's insurance?

Some transplant centers also include a pharmacist and a dietitian on the transplant team, who may also meet with you.

Transplant pharmacist. A pharmacist who specializes in working with people contemplating or undergoing organ transplants. This specialist works mainly with the kidney patient, whose post-transplant regimen will include antirejection medications, but also meets with the potential living donor and will advise on medication use.

Potential Questions: Will I need to take any medications because of having only one kidney? What prescription or over-the-counter medications will I need to avoid after donating? Will I need to stop any drugs before surgery, such as oral contraceptives?

Transplant dietitian. A dietitian or nutritionist who specializes in working with organ transplant patients and who also advises living donors on nutrition and weight loss. If a potential donor is overweight or obese, depending on body mass index (BMI), the dietitian will sometimes design a weight loss and nutrition program to help him or her become eligible to donate.

Potential Questions: Are there any particular foods I'll need to avoid with just one kidney? Which foods are good to eat if you have just one kidney? If I regain much of the weight that I shed for the donor surgery, will the weight affect me more now that I will have only one kidney?

CHAPTER 7

In-Depth Donor Evaluation

AT THIS POINT, THE DONOR COORDINATOR will arrange a full day or two of testing and meetings with all or most of the transplant team members. Remember, most of them are specifically assigned to *you* and will not interact with the recipient.

Carol's full day of interviews and initial appointments in her donor evaluation entailed meeting with most of the transplant team members plus having (1) a blood draw that took more than a dozen tubes of blood for lab work, (2) a chest X-ray, and (3) an EKG. Also, she took home a large container and a collection receptacle for a twenty-four-hour urine collection.

BASIC TESTS FOR MOST DONORS

Depending on your age, sex, and health conditions, you will take all or most of the tests below. We have listed the popular name first; the clinical term is in parentheses.

CT Scan (computed tomography angiogram)

What: A low-radiation 3-D scan.

Why: To provide detailed images of the donor's blood vessels and organs and to help the surgeon decide which kidney to take for the donation. (The left kidney is preferred because the vein is longer, which makes it easier to remove from you and to implant in the recipient's body.)

How: You lie on a narrow table that slides into the center of a ring-shaped scanner, which rotates around you to take the X-rays. To make the images clearer, you will have contrast dye injected through an IV. You may also be asked to swallow contrast dye if the surgeons want clearer detail of your intestines.

How long: About 20 minutes.

Renal Ultrasound

What: A painless, noninvasive test that uses sound waves instead of radiation to produce black-and-white images of the kidneys.

Why: To check the health, size, and location of your kidneys. It can also see kidney stones and blood flow in the kidneys. It is a good screening test to ensure that you have two normal-appearing kidneys of relatively equal size without kidney stones, cysts, or masses (tumors). Some centers perform this first to avoid the CT scan and IV contrast in anyone who does not have two healthy-appearing kidneys and therefore could not be a donor.

How: You lie on a regular examination table, and the technician first applies a gel to the area to make it easier to slide a small, hand-held wand called a *transducer* across your skin. The sound waves bounce off the organs and back to the transducer, and are converted into pictures.

How long: About half an hour to an hour.

EKG (or ECG, electrocardiogram)

What: Electrodes connected to you and a machine by wires painlessly measure the heart's electric activity.

Why: To detect a heart attack or, more commonly for a potential living donor, heart rhythm problems, such as an irregular heartbeat or a too-fast beat.

How: The electrodes are attached to small, plastic patches, which stick to your skin. They are placed on your chest, arms, and legs (yes, removal from hairy areas can hurt but only briefly). The EKG does not send electricity into the body.

How long: Only 5 to 10 minutes.

Chest X-Ray

What: A painless, standard X-ray of the chest—the most commonly performed diagnostic X-ray.

Why: To check for numerous abnormalities in a person's heart, lungs, and blood vessels, airways, and bones of the chest. It can detect underlying causes for common symptoms such as cough or shortness of breath.

How: You'll stand, sit, or lie still for the X-ray, with a lead apron in place to protect reproductive organs. It can be done at a clinic or hospital—even a doctor's office.

How long: 20 to 30 minutes.

Urine Test, 24-Hour Collection

What: A complete collection of urine during a 24-hour period.

Why: To measure kidney function; 24-hour collection measures volume and urine creatinine excretion, along with the amount of protein in the urine, allowing for a more accurate calculation of glomerular filtration rate (GFR) than a blood test alone. The urine and blood creatinine measurements, along with age, sex, and body size, are used to define kidney function. Too much protein spilling into the urine may be the earliest sign of kidney problems.

How: To collect urine at home, you'll use a special collection receptacle, which resembles an upside-down hat and rests on the toilet, and a container in which to pour the urine. Both items are provided by the transplant center or clinic.

How long: 24 hours.

Nuclear Medicine GFR Scan

What: An alternative test to a 24-hour urine collection to establish kidney function using nuclear medicine.

Why: This is much shorter, and even more accurate, than a 24-hour urine sample and can be done on-site at the hospital. It can also tell which of your kidneys is functioning better.

How: A radioactive dye is injected by IV into your arm. You sit under a camera, which measures the contrast that is absorbed by your kidneys and excreted by your kidneys. It can measure the total function of your kidneys, and tell how much is made by your left versus right kidney, which could be important if your kidneys appear to be different sizes. It can also tell if urine leaves one of your kidneys abnormally slowly (partial blockage).

How long? 4 hours.

ADDITIONAL STANDARD TESTS FOR CERTAIN DONORS

Depending on your age and sex, other tests may be required.

FOR LIVING DONORS OVER 50 YEARS OLD

Echocardiogram and/or Exercise Heart Stress Test

What: Sound waves (an ultrasound) create images of the heart's chambers and valves. At rest, this is called an echo. When the echo is taken before and during moderate to heavy exercise—that is, when the heart is stressed—it is an exercise stress test.

Why: To show problems in the heart's chambers or coronary arteries that supply blood to the heart, which sometimes occur only during physical activity.

How: The technician takes a preliminary reading while you lie on a table at rest; then you'll either walk on a treadmill or use a stationary bike. You'll be instructed to increase the intensity of the exercise and continue until you feel exhausted and can't continue. If you're on a bike, they'll take another reading during the exercise. In any case, they'll also take a reading immediately after the exercise.

How long: 45 minutes to an hour (the exercise part is only 7 to 12 minutes).

Colonoscopy (if you're up to date on the test, you simply provide documentation)

What: An examination of the entire large intestine (colon).

Why: To discover precancerous polyps, tumors, or other abnormalities that could jeopardize your health or make donation risky. (This is now suggested for all Americans starting at age 45.)

How: The physician uses a long, flexible tube that has a tiny camera and light on the end to view the colon. During the procedure you will be in a twilight sleep, which is much shorter-lived than general anesthesia but makes the procedure pain free for most people.

How long: 30 to 60 minutes.

FOR FEMALE LIVING DONORS

(Similarly, if you are up to date on these tests, simply provide documentation):

Pap Smear

What: It examines cells from a woman's cervix.

Why: To test for cervical cancer or precancerous changes.

How: A physician places a speculum inside the vagina and, using a swab, takes a sample of cells from the cervix.

How long: 10 to 15 minutes.

Mammogram

What: A low-dose X-ray of breast tissue.

Why: To detect cysts and tumors that are too small to be identified through physical examination.

How: A machine uses hard, clear plastic plates to apply pressure, flattening the breast as much as possible, to ensure a clear image before taking the X-ray.

How long: About 10 to 15 minutes; there is additional waiting time while the technician checks to see if any of the views need to be redone. The radiologist may or may not examine the films the same day.

POSSIBLE SPECIALIZED TESTS

After the transplant nephrologist and surgeon examine the test results and meet with you to explain the procedure and the risks, they may order still more tests.

MRI (magnetic resonance imaging)

Sometimes, when a donor's test results show irregularities or abnormalities and further tests are still inconclusive, the physicians may recommend an MRI. Certain abnormalities are easier to clarify by one imaging technique than another.

What: A noninvasive test using a magnetic field and radio waves to create detailed, often 3-D, images of organs and tissues.

Why: Its high-resolution images can identify tumors and other abnormalities in organs, tissues, and the skeletal system.

How: You lie very still in a long, narrow, tube-shaped machine (essentially a giant magnet), and a contrast dye is injected through an IV line to enhance the clarity of the pictures. People with claustrophobia should discuss this in advance with the doctor or technician and might be given sedation beforehand. While the machine moves, it produces a very loud, ongoing banging sound; you will be provided with earplugs or earbuds for music to shut out the noise.

How long: 30 minutes to an hour.

Lung (Pulmonary) Function Test

Similarly, because Carol's chest X-ray results were suspicious for a non-smoker, she next had a lung function test.

What: A noninvasive test that measures how well your lungs work—specifically, how much air your lungs can hold and how quickly they can push out the air. It can also measure how well gases go across your lung tissue and into your blood. Sometimes a blood gas test is also done to determine the amount of oxygen and carbon dioxide.

Why: To ensure that you can safely undergo general anesthesia for surgery. This test also can check whether your lung function improves with asthma inhalers.

How: Using a special mouthpiece connected to a spirometer, an instrument that takes the readings, you will be told to breathe rapidly and/or deeply (while your nose is closed with a clip); sometimes, the test is done while the person sits in an airtight glass box that looks like a small telephone booth.

How long: About 45 minutes.

ABPM (ambulatory blood pressure monitoring)

If you have high blood pressure readings during the evaluation and were not known to have high blood pressure, 24-hour monitoring will provide more accurate, comprehensive information.

What: A way of measuring your blood pressure while you go about normal activities.

Why: To get multiple readings in different situations, which provide a more complete picture, free of "white coat hypertension"—that is, higher blood pressure readings that sometimes result from a person's anxiety in a doctor's office.

How: You wear a blood pressure cuff on your arm, which is attached to a small recording device on your belt; it takes continuous blood pressure readings 'round the clock.

When all of the testing is complete, the transplant coordinator will review all of the donor testing with the Living Donor Selection Committee. If approved, you will be given the green light for the surgery. The donor coordinator will give you the news and may offer you additional time to think over your decision. If you want to go ahead, the surgery will be scheduled several weeks in advance, based on both the recipient's and your own needs and the surgeons' schedules. With few exceptions, the donor surgery and the transplant will be performed at the same time, often in adjacent operating rooms.

REPEATING A FEW TESTS BEFORE SURGERY

Cross-Matching

When: You usually give a blood sample at the transplant hospital, or it may be sent in by mail if you live far away, within two weeks of the actual transplant surgery.

Why: The recipient's antibody levels may have changed since last tested, as a result of infections, blood transfusions, miscarriages, or even minor surgeries.

Chest X-Ray

When: About a week before surgery.

Why: To ensure that you have not contracted any new infections.

Lab Work

When: About a week before surgery.

Why: To ensure that you have not contracted any new infections or ones that were not detected earlier, and to recheck your blood count, as well as have a specimen available in case you need a blood transfusion—very rare for the donor.

CHAPTER 8

"D" Day at Last!

YOU WILL PROBABLY CHECK INTO the hospital early, about 6 a.m., on the day of the donation; the recipient may be admitted the day before. The donor coordinator will greet you and review everything. Even at this late point, you may again be asked if you are certain about going ahead with the donation. The anesthesiologist will meet with you that morning even if you have already met during the pre-op appointment.

The donor surgery takes three to four hours, and your hospital stay will usually be one or two days. If you are an out-of-town donor, the transplant center may suggest that you stay in the area for one to two weeks. Initially, you will probably feel worse than the recipient. Yes, you've both just had major surgery, but remember, you're a healthy person who's had an organ removed, whereas your recipient has just received a healthy kidney that already works far better than the old one(s). Also, your surgery usually entails manipulating the intestines to get to your kidney, whereas the recipient's can be done without directly bothering the intestines. Your recovery will proceed faster than the recipient's, though, and your hospital stay will be shorter.

Pain management is handled in a variety of ways depending on the transplant center. Many centers have limited their use of a self-administered, but regulated, pain medication pump for donors as part of efforts to combat the opioid epidemic. Instead, they combine different types of pain medications to decrease the amount of narcotics required to control the pain. They may start some of them just before and during surgery.

The pump is often still used for the first day after surgery and has the advantage of eliminating the need to call a nurse to request the drugs—and yes, you may need them at first.

On the day after surgery, your urinary catheter will be removed (that takes less than a minute), and by the next day, you will begin to regain your strength. The pain should be more manageable by then. Carol left the hospital with a prescription for a mild painkiller, which she used for just a few days.

After the initial post-op period, which may require stool softeners and, possibly, anti-acid medication, you'll have no required medications related to donation. Minimizing the amount of narcotics used for the pain has the added benefit of allowing your bowels to wake up faster.

Probably the most common, though rare, surgical complication is the risk of a hernia at the site where the kidney is removed. This is often due to the donor's being too active soon after surgery. As with any surgery inside the abdomen, there is also a small risk of bowel obstruction.

Transplant centers are now required to do donor follow-ups at six months, one year, and two years. After that, just an annual check-up by your own provider, to include kidney function and blood pressure, takes care of the only long-term monitoring needed.

As is typical of surgery with a general anesthesia, it may take four to six weeks to completely lose the lingering fatigue. Carol enjoyed taking afternoon naps for a few weeks, which she recalls as the most satisfying, guilt-free naps of her life.

Scars from the tiny incisions virtually disappear over time, and the three-inch bikini incision (or just below the navel) will usually fade considerably with each passing year. For most living kidney donors, the fading scar is the only physical reminder of the donation. The pride, however, lasts a lifetime.

Part Two:
Our Stories

CHAPTER 9

Why (and How)
I Donated My Kidney

I MUST HAVE GONE THROUGH all that testing and even the surgery, but I have no idea how. You see, there's one aspect of living donation that you rarely hear much about. It even feels a bit unseemly to bring up when talking about something as crucial as saving a life. But I strongly suspect I'm not the only one to ever feel this way, so I want to raise it here at the beginning of my story.

The truth is, I'm a wimp when it comes to anything medical or physical. If my college yearbook had had a category for "Least Likely to Be a Living Kidney Donor," that would have been me. I've been known to faint at a flu shot, and once I passed out in anticipation of a blood test that never even happened. Much like my friend Linda—who not only wanted an epidural for childbirth, but wanted to be put under in her eighth month—I would have welcomed the idea of being put under for the first blood test only to awaken six months later minus one kidney. But my son, Paul, had kidney failure. Naturally, I had to be evaluated as a donor—and awake at that. Fortunately for me, early on I found a support system in the transplant team, which held my hand and, incredibly, never made me feel foolish or cowardly. More about that later.

For most families with a loved one contemplating a kidney transplant, the situation evolves over several years. People with polycystic kidney disease (PKD), like Betsy and her sisters (see Betsy's story, next chapter), may have lived with the threat for decades. Our family had just a few weeks to absorb a series of frightening revelations: Paul's kidneys suddenly appeared to be failing; he would soon need dialysis; he first had to have vascular surgery to put in an access point—and, ultimately, he would need a kidney transplant.

No wonder that all of us (my husband, Neil; our almost-fifteen-year-old daughter, Nora; Paul; and I) were reeling.

To be clear, the news wasn't entirely out of left field. A few years before, when Paul was in college, he was diagnosed with IgA nephropathy, a form of nephritis (an inflammation of the kidneys that affects kidney function). We had no family history, and he had none of the usual risk factors like diabetes or hypertension. What he had was a lingering strep infection, a not uncommon cause. The nephritis was discovered in lab work. Because he had no symptoms and was otherwise healthy, the nephrologist said it was something important to monitor but might never advance. If it did, it could conceivably take twenty years, he assured us. And surely by then, modern medicine would have found a successful treatment, if not a cure.

Paul had regular lab work throughout college. When the level of his creatinine (the chemical waste product in the blood that reflects how well the kidneys are functioning) started to edge up, the nephrologist sent Paul to a specialist and ordered a biopsy. The results weren't conclusive, so Paul continued to be monitored and was put on megadoses of fish oil in an attempt to slow the decline. Though it certainly concerned all of us, we tried to focus on the positive.

The Shock

Then, one day a couple of months after Paul's college graduation, his routine lab work revealed that his creatinine level had shot up—so much so that his nephrologist suspected a fluke and wanted to retest him. This time I accompanied Paul to the appointment. There the nephrologist not only confirmed the initial results but said Paul's creatinine was even higher now. To this day, no one knows what caused this precipitous rise. For an hour, Paul and I heard words like *dialysis, vascular access, fistula, catheter, transplant, organ donors* through a fog. Some of the terms were vaguely familiar but with ominous overtones, and some we'd never heard before. Still, we could barely ask questions—we were too dazed.

The timing could not have been worse for a young man who already had to contend with significant daily stressors. For much of his life Paul has struggled with obsessive compulsive disorder, marked by a fear of germs so strong that his hands are perpetually red and raw from frequent washing. His prolonged routines make scheduling very difficult. Paul had just graduated from college after six challenging but immensely enjoyable and gratifying years. Now that his perseverance and conscientiousness had been rewarded with a degree in math, he was eager to begin his life as an adult, get a real job, a new apartment. All of those plans and hopes were dashed in the space of that hour.

When I went home and told Neil and Nora the news, at first we just sat in silence. I don't remember who was the first to break the long silence by saying the words we were all thinking: "I want to be tested as a donor." I remember the shock at hearing my own words. Did I really say that? Nora said it too. Even though we were extremely proud of her, to our immense relief the transplant team wouldn't consider her as a potential donor because she was under eighteen. The thought of both our children undergoing major surgery at the same time was more than we could bear.

The next step, we soon learned, was to schedule surgery to provide a vascular access for the hemodialysis: a fistula connecting the artery and vein in Paul's arm. We lived the next few months in a state of suspended animation as we raced the clock, hoping that the surgery could be scheduled soon, be successful, and allow sufficient time for the fistula to "mature" before it was needed for dialysis, a process that could take six to eight weeks. Also, we were told there was only a 40% chance that the surgery would succeed. Consequently, Paul was facing the alarming possibility of needing a catheter in his neck for the dialysis if he were to reach that point without a functioning fistula. The worse-than-even odds of success for the fistula must have felt particularly unfair when he was still reeling from the initial news. He was so depressed that we worried he might not have the emotional strength to tackle this newest challenge given that there wasn't even a hint of light at the end of this long, winding tunnel. Somehow, he managed to trudge on.

At least one of us—usually me, because my job offered more flexibility than Neil's—attended all of Paul's appointments: nephrologist, vascular access coordinator, vascular access surgeon, the transplant team … Naturally, I missed a lot of work but fortunately was able to mostly work from home. On the phone one day, choking back tears, I told my supervisor that I couldn't bear to see or talk to colleagues in person. I wouldn't know what to say in response to well-meaning remarks like "How's your son?" "I hope he's doing better." "Hope he gets better soon." No, he wasn't "better," he wouldn't be better for a very long time, and things would surely get considerably worse before they could even begin to get better. Not the sort of thing you want to repeat or hear throughout your workday.

Similarly, Neil and I began to avoid social situations. When someone says "How've you been?" and really wants to know, you can't just say "Oh, fine" (well, *I* couldn't—Neil managed that a lot better than I did)—nor can you repeat the whole story over and over at a group gathering. So we socialized mostly with close friends who already knew the situation. And if I spotted someone in a store whom I hadn't seen in a long time, I'd duck behind a tall display and hope the person hadn't seen me.

As Paul's creatinine continued to rise, we prayed that dialysis could wait long enough. Thankfully, for once (as Paul would say) he got lucky: the access surgery succeeded beautifully, and the fistula was up and running by the time he got the word to start dialysis about two months later.

During this time, Neil and I were filling out long evaluation forms as the first step in the donor screening. Neil didn't make the first cut because of a kidney stone a few years before. My sister and brother-in-law, who volunteered, never even got that far: they were both the wrong blood type—we needed type O, the universal donor, because Paul was type O. (Paired donation, now common, in which you can "swap" donors in such cases, wasn't even on our radar at the time.)

Dialysis

Given the very real possibility that I would eventually be Paul's donor, with my wimp background in mind, I had to wonder if I really could do this. I figured I'd better get to work on making it possible and decided to tackle *observing* dialysis. My first visit to the center where Paul would later have his dialysis was a relative success: I didn't pass out. Of course, I also didn't allow myself to gaze at anything for long.

Once Paul started dialysis, however, I began to force myself to watch when the technician inserted the needle. In fact, I paid close attention and attended every dialysis session in the first few months. Obsessively keeping detailed records, I filled steno notebooks with numbers that quantified a brand-new vocabulary: needle size, flow, dry weight (his target weight without the extra fluid that builds up between dialysis sessions). I took some small comfort in having something to compare, however opaque it all was. I also recorded some familiar numbers: Paul's pre- and post-dialysis blood pressure readings, plus the readings recorded during the session. I won't pretend that I understood it all, but having a professional editor's eye for detail served me well: I just watched for inconsistencies. When a reading differed sharply from his usual numbers, I watched all the more closely. Occasionally, it was far more obvious, like a needle inserted improperly and blood trickling down his arm.

Previously, I'd thought of dialysis as a fairly straightforward process. I soon learned and marveled that a complex art was required to find the right balance of fluids and nutrients. Paul had to strictly watch his diet to keep the right proportions of potassium and sodium and phosphorus, a task that would have just been part of a day's work for healthy kidneys. One day at dialysis, a technician apparently made a bad call on the goal for Paul's dry weight, and his blood pressure consequently shot up to well over 200. Distressed, the next day I related the incident to the nephrologist who was the center director. He was suitably concerned and told me that if I ever again suspected a mistake, or had a concern, to call him at home. I tried not to abuse the privilege but did have occasion to call him a few times. I never saw that tech again and assume she was fired. I liked her, and it wasn't like me to "report" someone, but I was learning a new boldness in my advocacy role, and I soon got over any pangs of guilt.

I made it through the first round in the evaluation, but the hospital wouldn't allow me to begin the actual testing because Paul did not have health insurance that would cover my costs. It's customary for the recipient's health insurance to pay for the donor's testing, which at the time could have easily run to $10,000 per donor (it's now potentially as high as $15,000). Because Paul was no longer a full-time student, he was not covered by our family's health insurance. (Note that this was before the Affordable Care Act was passed in 2010, which would have allowed Paul, then under twenty-six, to remain on our family's plan.) Instead, he had Medicaid, which also typically pays for the donor. However, as of just a month before, because of North Carolina state cutbacks, Medicaid had stopped paying for the donor's expenses. Ironically, Medicare actually has an ESRD (end-stage renal disease) category, which should have covered it (and ultimately did). But, in a classic Catch-22, Paul, fresh out of college and in poor health, had not yet worked long enough to accrue sufficient credits to qualify. It's not hard to understand why Paul felt that the cards were stacked against him at times.

After reflexively volunteering to be Paul's donor, I'll admit I was beginning to waver a bit—and not just because of needles. We had recently moved my then-ninety-year-old father down from New York to our town, and though he did not live with us, I was his primary caregiver. I hired and oversaw his home health aides, accompanied him to doctor visits, handled his finances, had power of attorney—all the while working full time. In addition, Nora, by then sixteen, was struggling through a rough patch in adolescence. A very bright kid who later aced the SATs, she came close to failing more than one subject that school year. Neil and I recognized that we'd both been preoccupied with our son's condition and the responsibilities of my father's care, and felt certain that this situation had inevitably contributed to Nora's difficulties, a fact she continues to deny to this day.

For me, the stress of parenting and eldercare was often overwhelming. I'll never forget the time a delay with my son at his nephrologist appointment made me pick my dad up late for his cardiologist appointment that same morning. After laboriously getting Dad in and out of the car and wheelchair, through the lobby, and up in the elevator, we were fifteen minutes late for his appointment. The receptionist coolly told us that because the cardiologist had to leave soon she couldn't see him, and we'd have to reschedule. I burst into tears. (It didn't help.) Another time I ran out of one of my dad's urologist appointments, leaving him to wait alone for the driver from his new assisted-living facility to pick him up, so I could get Paul to dialysis on time.

When I described our family situation to the donor social worker, she asked if my plan to be Paul's donor was realistic, or at least wise. "You're the glue that's holding it all together," she said. "What happens when you're not available, when *you* need care—even if it's only for a limited time?" It was a valid question, and it nagged at me for a long time. How would Neil be able to care for Paul, Nora, my father, and me too? I didn't know the answer, but I took a few small concrete steps. I explained the situation to the director of my father's assisted living facility, pointing out that I couldn't be filling in the gaps in care as I usually did. Naturally, she told me I had nothing to worry about concerning his care—a dubious reassurance, but it felt comforting at the time. I also contacted the realtors who were selling our townhouse (Paul's diagnosis came on the heels of our family's move). Fortunately, we trusted them implicitly to arrange for repairs and refurbishing, so it was a no-brainer to just let them run with it.

Dialysis continued to dominate Paul's life and sap his strength, both physically and emotionally. Three days a week for three hours at a time he was tethered to a machine. With prep time and post-time, plus another hour for transportation, it was well over half a day—not to mention the fatigue that invariably followed. He had time and energy for little else. Although he handled the tedium and the rules fairly resourcefully, the perception of being unclean was almost intolerable for him. He would go straight home and take long showers after every session. Also, he felt like a prisoner under house arrest. The only way that travel far from home was possible was through elaborate arrangements with another dialysis center wherever he might want to go—assuming there was one. He couldn't skip a dialysis session without a compelling reason, and then would have to arrange a special schedule outside his regular slot. I remember feeling guilty when the rest of the family spent a week at the beach without Paul, after trying in vain to figure out a way to get him there and back between sessions.

And year-round, we all lived in dread of bad weather: snow, icy roads, thunderstorms, power outages—anything that could jeopardize transportation to and from the dialysis center or even threaten the services themselves. What if the center had a power outage? Or the technicians couldn't get to work? Or if Paul were sick and couldn't go for dialysis?

Not surprisingly, Paul thought about nothing but the transplant and being freed from the burden of dialysis. At every checkup, he greeted the nephrologist with lots of questions about the transplant. To his credit, the doctor patiently went into great detail about things that Paul, alas, wouldn't face for nearly two more years because of the delay in getting Medicare.

One of the important ways that Paul prepared for the transplant was to learn to swallow pills. We were told that after the transplant he would come home from the hospital on a regimen of more than thirty pills a day, most of which could not be chewed, crushed, or compounded like his usual meds. Paul had a very strong gag reflex, and when he was a child, we'd tried every trick possible, even putting a pill in a marshmallow. One of the great achievements that made the transplant possible resulted from work at the hospital's swallowing disorders clinic, which helps stroke patients and others relearn how to swallow. Neil and I both attended the first few sessions and watched in awe as the skilled therapist worked creatively with Paul. He even devised homework for him to practice with small chunks of ice, to minimize his gag reflex. Once that happened, we knew Paul would be able to make progress.

The Green Light for Testing

Meanwhile, for more than a year we made countless phone calls and wrote pleading letters to the hospital, insurance companies, state agencies, our congressman, the state Ombud's program, and donor organizations. Thanks to the continued and passionate advocacy of the hospital's transplant nephrologists, the hospital finally agreed to shoulder the costs if Medicare did not come through in time and gave the green light for me to begin the testing. Excitedly, I began a full schedule of appointments and interviews: with a transplant nurse coordinator, my social worker, my psychologist, my transplant nephrologist, my transplant surgeon. Yes, all mine, to support *me*. I loved having a professional I could talk to about my concerns or questions 24/7 both before and after the transplant. Everyone assured me that if I were to change my mind at any point, Paul need never know. He would just be told that I was eliminated. For much of the testing period, the transplant team was short staffed, so Paul and I had the same nurse coordinator. I can honestly say, though, that I never felt any pressure from her. Liz skillfully and thoughtfully managed to support both of us based on our own distinct needs.

Knowing my wimp history, Liz gently helped me through the testing process. She had the lab take as many tubes of blood as possible at once to avoid their needing to stick me extra times—fortunately, she didn't tell me they would take more than a dozen at one appointment. She advised me to apply lidocaine to numb my arm in advance of a blood draw—we even experimented with different prescription strengths. That was an enormous help.

After each battery of tests, I'd call her at the appointed time—from a day to a week later—and hold my breath till I learned if I'd passed. Even after months of successful testing, I knew that I could still be eliminated. How would I feel? Would I secretly be relieved? (Hey, I tried.) Much to my surprise, I realized that I'd be crushed. I wanted to be the one to free Paul from this long nightmare. I also wanted to prove to myself that I could do it, that I could meet a physical challenge, conquer one of my biggest fears. I'd always striven to stretch myself mentally, socially, professionally—but never before physically.

Also, if I couldn't donate to Paul, we had no Plan B—no one else had come forward. Because Paul could receive an organ only from a type O donor, in North Carolina that meant he might have to wait an additional five years or more for a deceased donor, with not nearly as good a prognosis. Given that a live-donor kidney generally starts working immediately, Paul also wouldn't need to stay on dialysis waiting for it to start up. And when you add the increased chance of a live kidney lasting far longer, it became crystal-clear. I not only wanted to do this, I had to do it.

At last, I cleared the final hurdle: I "passed," and the surgeon confirmed that he could do my surgery laparoscopically. Although that is now the standard of care for donor nephrectomies, there are still some rare situations that make it too challenging. We scheduled the surgery for a few weeks later. I was giddy with excitement—and, of course, panic at the thought of major surgery. What was that intense pounding in my chest—was I having palpitations? And suddenly it seemed so hard to take a deep breath. Surely that wasn't normal. One of the many evaluations I had was a pulmonary function test, in which

I had to blow into a tube as hard as possible. To help prevent postoperative pneumonia, a patient needs to be able to breathe deeply. Could I?

I shared my concerns with Ann, my new nurse coordinator. When I described the situation, she listened sympathetically and promised to talk to the surgeons. A few minutes later, Ann called back to say that they had assured her my heart and lung function were both just fine. Perhaps I'd like to talk to the psychologist, she asked. Sure, why not?

When I explained my concerns to the psychologist, she surprised me by asking gently if I'd like to reschedule the surgery. *Ohmygod*, she thinks I'm having second thoughts! Nothing could have been further from the truth. "You don't understand," I told her. "I'd be the same if I were having my tonsils out."

Donation Day!

The big day finally arrived. Paul checked into the hospital the day before so he could have dialysis in the hospital. I had to get there the next morning by 6 a.m. Paul went into the operating room first to be prepped and then they got me ready in a nearby room. When they removed my kidney, they took it directly to his waiting body, where they tucked it inside his lower belly—for a total of three kidneys.

After my surgery, Neil and Nora came in to see me after seeing Paul, who'd emerged from the OR before me. They reported that when they asked him how he was, Paul's memorable, endearing answer was "Could be worse."

The transplant floor, unlike the rest of the hospital other than the maternity ward, is a relatively happy place. Most of these surgeries had been carefully scheduled, and the prospects for newfound health cautiously optimistic. Sounds of congratulations and good wishes filled the air. The floor nurses and other staff made me feel like a heroine, an experience I'd never had before or since. I was prepared for the relief and the satisfaction that followed the surgery, but not the incredible high.

Paul was in a great mood, too—we all were: a combination of relief and guarded excitement at the improvements to come. On that first night, what little sleep I had was tranquil, for the first time in years undisturbed by fears of what lay ahead. I knew Paul wasn't out of the woods yet, but for now I was content to take the first hurdle in stride, pat myself on the back, and say, "Job well done, Carol—I'm proud of you." Yup, I felt justifiably proud of myself, perhaps for the first time in my life. The only thing that marred that night was the phlebotomist's arrival every few hours for the blood draws. I sleepily tried to tell her that I was used to applying lidocaine first and waiting twenty to thirty minutes … Alas, she wasn't buying it.

For the first twenty-four hours or so, I was told to expect, the donor is in more pain than the recipient. Sure enough, Paul was able to walk to my room for a visit before I could walk to his. My nurse coordinator, Ann, pointed out that the surgeon had just put my healthy body through an ordeal, "tiptoeing" through my intestines to get to my kidney. To remove my kidney laparoscopically, the surgeon made two tiny slits near my belly button to insert minuscule cameras to guide the removal of the kidney, which was taken out through a three-inch bikini incision.

As Ann had predicted, my worst pain was actually near my shoulders ("referred pain" that travels along a nerve from the diaphragm muscle, which is irritated from the gas used during the surgery). It was a sharp pain that made me clutch at my shoulders. It hurt most when I laughed. Unfortunately my husband, whose wit has usually served to relieve tension, had a bad habit of making me laugh. Thanks to a marvelous push-button control, though, I could dispense my own pain meds with every laugh—and without having to fear overdosing. When they removed the catheter, and eventually the IV, after a day or two, I had my hand on that button whenever I needed. (Transplant centers are using the pumps less and less for donors now, as they look for alternative approaches to pain management in an effort to curb opioid abuse.) By the time I left the hospital on the fourth day, I needed only a mild painkiller. In fact, I remember the surgeon's good-natured admonishment the day before: "Why are you still in a gown? You're not sick!"

From the beginning, staff and visitors repeatedly told me how good I looked. True, I'd had a new haircut and joked that my hair stylist could list "pre-op hairdos" as a new specialty, but I don't think that's what they meant. They often said, "you don't seem like someone who just donated a kidney." I didn't feel like one either.

At Home

When my husband went to the pharmacy to pick up my pain medication, the pharmacist was clearly impressed that it was a particularly mild one. "She must be really tough," he said admiringly. Obviously, that was hardly the case. The pain simply wasn't as bad as I'd feared. When friends visited me at home, they were surprised to see me answer the door in street clothes. I remember talking to my cousin on the phone soon after being released from the hospital. She was delighted and taken aback to hear my strong voice as I readily picked up the house phone. She confessed that she'd pictured "something like round-the-clock nursing care." I was almost as surprised as everyone else, frankly. I felt so much better than I'd thought I would that I confided to a friend, only half-jokingly, that I almost wondered if they'd done it right.

Over the next few weeks and months, on meeting people for the first time I could sense a respect and even awe when they learned that I'd been a donor. That felt great, though it made me uncomfortable when someone would say, "you must be so brave." Bravery had nothing to do with it. I likened it to childbirth: we all know it's going to be painful, but we do it anyway. When I was a new mother, no one ever thought to mention my courage.

Other than the mild painkiller, my only meds in those first few weeks were for stomach acid and a laxative. My only dietary restrictions similarly were designed to ensure regular bowel movements. I have no ongoing dietary restrictions related to my kidney. It took a couple of weeks to get everything functioning efficiently again, but my discomfort was minimal. I walked regularly, enjoyed an afternoon nap when I got tired, and gradually resumed all my activities. I felt so good that I forgot about the rule against lifting anything heavier than six pounds during the post-op period and strained a bit to pick up a storage box before being scolded by my husband.

My own creatinine level, that critical number we'd watched climb so alarmingly for Paul in his pre-dialysis days, began its comforting descent. For most women, a reading of less than 1.2 is generally normal, and immediately post-transplant mine was predictably just borderline. Since then, as expected, it's gradually gone down (I hate to boast, but at a recent checkup, it was 0.75!).

Paul was released from the hospital a day after me. The plan was for him to recuperate at our home, so I fretted about making the house safe for him. To ensure that on the way to his room he wouldn't need to walk past the lovely get-well bouquet of flowers I'd received from my colleagues (a no-no for the fragile transplant recipient for the first few weeks), I quarantined them in the master bathroom. I was pretty pleased with my efforts to guarantee this extra level of germ-free security—until I discovered that Paul and Nora had unwittingly been sharing a toothbrush (Nora's) for days! I laugh when I recall it now, but at the time I was furious at both of them.

Avoiding the ER

If only fresh flowers and shared toothbrushes were all we'd had to worry about that week. A few days later Paul began to have unbearable pain. By evening it was so intense that he was distraught and inconsolable. He began gagging every time he tried to take the antirejection meds. We worried that his body would start rejecting my kidney. The only way he might get down the antirejection meds was to get on top of the pain, but of course he couldn't get the pain meds down either. We didn't know what to do. It was the weekend, and we'd been told to keep him out of the ER at all costs: it's the last place you want to be with a severely suppressed immune system. The situation felt hopeless. In our exhausted state, Neil and I were both in despair. We went into the next room and cried in each other's arms.

Fortunately, Nora and my sister Marion, who was staying with us for the transplant, continued to work with Paul. They took turns staying up throughout the night to help him with his meds every four hours. They somehow pulled it off, spoon-feeding him the meds mixed with ice cream, and he gradually calmed down and even managed to sleep a little.

First thing Monday morning, Neil and Marion took Paul to the transplant clinic to be examined. A sonogram and X-rays showed internal bleeding, but the cause was unknown. He'd need to have *exploratory emergency surgery*. All the words were chilling. When Marion called me with the news, she said Neil had told her to say I didn't need to come to the hospital. I shot back that unless he had a damn good reason that I didn't know about, there was no way I wasn't coming to the hospital. When Nora heard the situation, she fought back tears and said she was coming too. Unfortunately I wasn't allowed to drive yet, so we had to wait for what seemed like hours for a friend to drive us there.

After the surgery, Paul's surgeon came to tell us the good news—they'd stopped the bleeding—and the bad news: they still could not determine the cause. Though we were relieved that the bleeding was stopped, we were naturally alarmed at the realization that it might well recur. For the next few days, we watched as Paul's pulse (at about 115) and blood pressure (about 180 on top), remained frighteningly high. This time he was also more debilitated. We mentioned to the doctors that he'd done so much better after the transplant surgery, and they pointed out that he had been taking steroids at the time, which also partly accounted for his high spirits. They wanted to send him home as soon as possible for fear that he'd contract an infection in the hospital, but we resisted, remembering how terrified we were when his condition deteriorated at home the first time. Get his condition under control, we said, and then we'll take him home. So for several days we walked a tightrope, wanting to keep Paul in the hospital till his condition stabilized—and yet wanting to get him the hell out of there.

Luckily, Paul managed to not contract an infection. Once again, we brought him home to our house to begin his post-op recovery. He was more fragile this time, and we were all well aware of all that could go wrong. We were fortunate to still have Marion with us. Funny, she'd thought she was coming to cook, drive, and hold down the fort. Little did we all know that she'd quickly become a valued member of the "team," taking notes when she and Neil met with the doctors, spelling Neil so he could get some rest, and of course jumping in during that harrowing night when Paul couldn't get down his meds.

As predicted, Paul came home from the hospital with a regimen of some thirty pills a day. He had a huge weekly pill box with slots for morning, midday, dinnertime, and bedtime. Together we set up the pills, going down the list, taking turns at carefully calling out the long names, and cross-checking which ones had to be taken with a meal or separated by X number of hours from food, which ones had to be separated from certain other meds—a daunting task. The first time it took us well over an hour to set things up, and we all felt drained.

We relaxed by playing Taboo and had fun devising new rules for choosing partners: exactly four kidneys per team. That meant that neither Paul nor I could be on a team with anyone else. For instance, if I paired up with Marion, we'd be short one kidney; if Paul paired with Nora, they'd have one kidney too many.

Day by day Paul grew a little stronger, and with each doctor's appointment, one more invasive piece of "equipment" was removed: a stent one day, a catheter another (and, a couple of years later, even the fistula). Slowly, he began to regain his life and feel more like himself. The lab work was a couple of times a week at first, then weekly, every two weeks, three weeks, and eventually every four to six weeks. Each time his meds would be adjusted till they got the balance just right. Even today, that delicate balance enables Paul to take just enough immunosuppressants to prevent rejection while having enough protection so that he doesn't have to live in a bubble. In fact, he rarely gets sick.

Our Emotional Marathon

We often recalled the surgeon's advice to think of this journey not as a sprint but a marathon—that is, to learn to pace our emotions—because Paul was not out of the woods yet. The first year was fraught with minefields, doctors warned us. Every time something good happened, we tried not to let our guard down lest we be devastated by the next setback. Amazingly, a major setback never came. Paul, as we knew he would, became the model patient in terms of compliance with his medication schedule. Whenever he had a special event or problematic travel arrangements, he was always prepared.

Paul's life will always be troubled by potential hazards, and he'll always need to take extra precautions. We check expiration dates a lot more closely when we're preparing a meal for him, cancel our Sunday get-togethers if one of us is sick even with a cold. His immune system, far stronger than in those early days, will always be suppressed to keep it from rejecting my kidney. But for the most part, I think he's made his peace with his body, willing to accept this way of life because it is so far superior to the nearly two years of dialysis "torture."

And I don't miss my left kidney. My right one is healthy and plump, as it enlarged to take on its expanded role. My only long-term restrictions, to avoid injuring it, are to avoid heavy contact and extreme sports and NSAIDs, such as ibuprofen, which can damage the kidneys.

Proudest Day

That day in June 2006, when I gave Paul a little piece of myself, is still the proudest day of my life. I am obviously not a brave person, I am not an adventurous person. I have never won any major honors or awards. But on my wall is a framed Certificate of Appreciation, which reads as follows:

In honor and recognition of your priceless gift of kidney donation.
Your gift brings with it the opportunity for renewed health and well-being
and represents the highest form of love and compassion for others.

I choked up when I read it aloud the day that Ann, my donor coordinator, gave it to me. It's signed by my transplant surgeon, my transplant physician, and Ann—and had it been signed by the Nobel Prize committee, it could not have conferred more honor. Even now when I find myself losing self-confidence, I have only to glance at it and remind myself not to sweat the small stuff.

When I say I would do it again in a heartbeat, that's not hyperbole due to the fourteen-year distance. I also said it a week after the transplant, when I was still pretty sore.

CHAPTER 10

Why (and How)
I Received a Kidney

TRANSPLANTS AND LIVING DONATION WERE not something I'd ever given any thought to when I was younger. So you can imagine my surprise when I was diagnosed with polycystic kidney disease (PKD) at the age of thirty-five. Here I was thinking I was in outstanding health only to be told I had large cysts in my kidneys that would gradually impair my kidney functioning. I immediately thought, where did this come from and how did I not know I had PKD? I was a graduate student at the University of Wisconsin and had been living in Madison for the last three and a half years. As graduate students did in the '80s, I drank smoothie shakes in the morning, ate yogurt for lunch, and often snacked on all varieties of Wisconsin cheese through the day. In a nutshell (or should I say cheese curd?), I overdosed on dairy products and developed disturbing symptoms of cramping, bloating, and abdominal discomfort.

When I consulted a doctor, after showing me the abdominal ultrasound (which looked like a mass of black holes in my kidneys), he gave me the shocking news that I had PKD. He also said I would forever need to be careful about car accidents and participating in any activities that might injure my kidneys—not the message a thirty-five-year-old "healthy," active person wants to hear.

That evening when I called to tell my mother, a Depression-era parent who did not believe in talking about illness, she matter-of-factly said, "Oh, yes, I have that too and I've never had those kinds of abdominal symptoms, so tell them to keep looking for the real cause." I was stunned that my own mother had PKD and, unbelievably, had never thought to mention it to me or my sisters. She made light of it to such an extent that I was lulled into thinking it must not be a very big deal. That was my first mistake, not to ask more questions or to dig deeper into my (and her) disease. My mother did say that PKD had never caused her any trouble, although she had to take medication for high blood pressure, which is often associated with kidney disease.

Because there was no Internet back then, I went to the library and was surprised to find so little information available to help me understand the disease. I was so uninformed, in fact, that the next year when I took a job that offered employer-sponsored life insurance, I instead chose to apply for an outside policy with better coverage. To my surprise, I was turned down because of my PKD and of course by then had missed the open enrollment for life insurance at my workplace. That was when I began to discover more about the potential long-term consequences of PKD. For example, as the insurance company was no doubt well aware and I would learn later, half of people with PKD will need dialysis or a kidney transplant at some point in their lifetime. Clearly, the lack of information was an early stumbling block for me that led to missteps in watching out for myself long term.

My (and My Family's) History

I began to ask more questions of my family members. I found out that my maternal grandmother had always had kidney "problems" but was never on dialysis or had a transplant. Her father, my maternal great-grandfather, had what was then called Bright's disease, a broad term for kidney disease. He died of kidney disease, probably PKD we know now. In my immediate family, I already knew that my oldest sister, Christie, had had a mass in one of her kidneys in her twenties and that her kidney had to be removed. At the time there was no real explanation—her doctor just said it had stopped functioning and become enlarged. Looking back some years later, we realized that it must have been PKD, and she just hadn't been diagnosed yet—nor had my mother. Among the four siblings in my family, three of us had PKD and all three of us had transplants in our fifties. My mother, who lived until she was eighty-two, only began to have end-stage renal failure in the last year of her life, so you can see why she had been unconcerned about having the disease. Her death was from other complications—none of them kidney related.

My sister Christie was the first to receive a transplant. In 2001 she gratefully received a kidney from her son, Andy, who used the experience to become healthier by slimming down and beginning to exercise more. They both continue to do well nineteen years later. Another of my sisters, Barbara, also had PKD and received a transplant in 2007. Unfortunately, she had many complications before and after her transplant, with diabetes and fibromyalgia in addition to heart and lung issues, and passed away in 2012 at the age of sixty-three. My third sister, Martha, is the lucky one and does not have PKD and is in good health.

My own history included many years of good health following my diagnosis in 1986, except for the eventual need to take medication for my rising blood pressure and unrelated lactose intolerance. In the fall of 2002, when my nephrologist of many years moved into full-time research and decided not to see patients anymore, I was referred to one of his colleagues, a much younger nephrologist. I was surprised at our first meeting that she recommended an MRI to check on my kidney status, but I assumed that she must just be very thorough and didn't give it a second thought.

To be quite honest, at that time I still wasn't following my "numbers"—mainly my creatinine, which shows the level of waste products in the blood, and GFR (kidney function)—so I wasn't aware that they were getting worse. Because the amount of protein in your urine can be a sign of kidney disease, as I later learned, paying attention to your albumin-to-creatinine ratio and your GFR is key to monitoring your kidney health. You may be thinking by now that I was a bit cavalier about the whole thing, but remember, my mother had done well into her eighties and only one of my sisters, Christie, had received a transplant by then. And given that Christie had only one kidney at the time, I just thought her transplant was an anomaly in the family. Barbara at the time, like me, was doing well even with her PKD, so transplants and dialysis were far from my mind.

You can understand my astonishment then when my new doctor started talking about the MRI results and moved immediately into talking about dialysis and eventual transplant. I will never forget that day when I went back to my office to try to work—all I could think about was the big "T" word she had mentioned, which I had not even thought a possibility (much less an eventuality) for me. In trying to understand how this had crept up on me, and without my previous doctor having discussed the decline in my numbers, I asked her how long it had been going on. She was very diplomatic in discussing my decline, especially given that my previous nephrologist had been one of her mentors. She noted that there were many differences between older and younger doctors and most particularly as to what and when information is shared with patients. As she explained, older doctors were often trained to shield their patients from "bad news" and generally only to share what they felt was critical at that time. In other words, my previous doctor, in feeling he was protecting me, had not shared my declining numbers because he did not want to upset me needlessly until the time that there was some action to take. My new doctor, on the other hand, was trained to partner with the patient in being able to jointly make healthcare decisions "with" and not "for" the patient. Her approach was to inform the patient as early as possible so that there would be true collaboration in these decisions. What an eye opener for me and what a refreshing attitude toward one's patients. Needless to say, that day I began to be a religious follower of my numbers so I could help monitor my own situation and never again be caught unaware. In addition, my doctor immediately referred me to a transplant surgeon (Dr. Andreoni, as it turned out) so that I could be as informed about the process as possible.

Unfortunately, to this day some nephrologists still do not know how helpful it is to refer their patients to a transplant program even before they may need dialysis. That way, if you have a living donor, there's time to have the donor go through testing and you may be able to have a transplant before you need to start dialysis. And if you do not have a living donor, you can start looking for one while being listed on the national deceased-donor waiting list (once your kidney function drops to 20% or lower). You begin accruing wait time, and it may be years before you need to start dialysis. You could even receive a deceased-donor transplant before having to start dialysis.

Getting Ready for a Double Nephrectomy

Over the next year, as my numbers got worse and I began to have a series of urinary tract infections (UTIs), we began to talk more seriously about dialysis and transplant. I was not opposed to dialysis and realized it was likely that I would have to do it at some point. My preference was to go ahead and identify a donor so that the transplant could take place as soon as possible. As my numbers declined significantly, I began to work with Dr. Andreoni who, like my new nephrologist, believed in informing his patients as early as possible and working with them in the planning process. He felt that given the new technologies in antibody matching, my husband, Mike, could potentially be a good donor for me. The surgeon also said that his surgical approach would be to take out both my kidneys in the first surgery (double nephrectomy), give me four months to recuperate, and then do the transplant. His rationale was that with my native kidneys filling with cysts, their numbers declining, and their causing frequent UTIs, I would be better off without them. Sometimes surgeons leave in the old kidney(s) and just add the new one. That's what happened with my older sister (and Carol's son, Paul, after her donation), but a few years later when my sister's remaining native kidney began to malfunction, they had to take it out. So, I actually thought getting rid of both of my native kidneys at once was a better idea.

Therefore, with the hope of Mike as my donor, I made plans that fall for handling my university teaching duties, so I would be ready for the surgery right after Thanksgiving. As Mike and I began to meet with various healthcare providers that made up his team—psychologists, nurses, doctors—he began the testing phase to find out whether he could be my donor. In addition to listing it on the health form, at least twice during the early phases we reported that Mike had had melanoma on his shoulder years before. Both the professionals we told assured us that the melanoma would not be a problem, but unfortunately it ultimately was. After completing all the testing, the last step was to meet with the transplant surgeon assigned to him (not the one working with me, to avoid a conflict of interest). This physician told us that if Mike were my donor there was a risk of my contracting some type of cancer, not necessarily melanoma, and that it would be Mike's and my decision whether to go through with the transplant.

Of course we were devastated at this news, and angry that during the months-long process no one had recognized this risk and talked with us about it. On the way home that day, I told Mike there was no way we could go through with our plan, because we would be putting us both at risk for cancer and we couldn't do that to our children. The next day someone from my surgeon's office called to say that the surgeon representing my husband had misspoken, and that they would not approve a transplant from my husband because of his melanoma. They then sent us a couple of journal articles about two recipients who had contracted cancer after each of them received a kidney from a deceased man who had had some type of previous cancer. Thus, as we read more it became clear that there was an increased risk of my getting cancer from Mike's kidney, so we knew we were not going to take that chance.

Of course, Mike and I were both crushed. The next few days at our house were pretty miserable as Mike and I struggled with what had happened and how to tell the kids. The hardest part of all of it was that the whole health-care team had been so positive about Mike being my donor that honestly, we didn't even consider a different outcome. In addition, when we had brought up his cancer early in the process, their many assurances had buoyed our hopes. To be fair, perhaps someone mentioned that we should not assume Mike could be a donor, but I surely don't remember anyone giving us the impression that he was likely to be ineligible. In fact, when we asked about Mike's chances, most of the professionals talked about the new antibody technologies and how many more people could be donors than in previous times. I do wish someone had made a point to caution us, so that we wouldn't have been so disappointed by the bad news. Telling the kids that Mike couldn't be my donor was one of the hardest things I've ever done. On one level, I think they might have been relieved that they wouldn't have to worry about him undergoing surgery too, but they were quite afraid for what was going to happen to me. Of course, we assured them that there had to be another donor out there somewhere and we would do our best to find one.

You can bet that after I, as the recipient, started getting the first bills for Mike's testing, I called the billing office as well as my surgeon and the transplant team. I wanted them to know that we would only pay the bills for the first visit or two, given that we had fully disclosed Mike's melanoma from the beginning and should have been told much sooner about this important risk.

They ultimately must have decided that we had an excellent case, because we did not get any further bills, and they actually cancelled the first few. It wasn't exactly our idea of a fair trade for what we went through, but at least they didn't expect my insurance to pay for their terrible mistake in missing this serious contraindication!

By this time it was early fall, and because I was continuing to have multiple UTIs, Mike and I, the surgeon, and my nephrologist decided to go ahead with the nephrectomy in November. Otherwise, there was the concern that I might end up being too sick to have the transplant. You can imagine that I was a bit apprehensive about having my kidneys removed when I didn't have a confirmed donor. But my optimism and my doctor's and my family's assurances that I would find a donor (not to mention that I was getting sicker) propelled me to get on with it. And then on my birthday, October 28, a very close cousin, Cindy Thomas, called to say she had a great birthday present for me: "Well, how about a kidney?" she said. Such a surprise and relief to think that I had at least one potential donor, but as I had already learned, I wasn't going to count any eggs until they hatched.

In the meantime, the university newspaper had written a story about me and my need for a donor. After the story appeared, several people volunteered to be donors: a woman I had known years before when I saw her young child for speech-language therapy, a former student who had been in our program, and even two complete strangers. I was incredibly shocked, relieved, and grateful. At the same time, a colleague, Laurie Cochenour, had volunteered and started donor testing only to find out she could not be a donor for me. In addition, a man I hardly knew, who was a chef at a favorite restaurant of ours at a vacation resort we frequented, also volunteered. When I found out he did not have any health insurance, however, even though my insurance would have paid his bills for the donation, I told him I couldn't possibly accept his offer because he would never get insurance later with only one kidney—this was before the Affordable Care Act (ACA). Given the uncertainty about coverage in today's healthcare climate, if you're considering donating, it's wise to check your own health insurance policy and that of any potential recipient before moving ahead. I hope not many people who need a kidney or want to donate one will be constricted by having to consider their accessibility to good health insurance, but at this time it's important to double-check. Also consider life insurance, because it is much more difficult to get affordable life insurance if you have one kidney or ESRD or PKD. The uncertainty about both health and life insurance is the reason our adult son and daughter have been advised not to get tested for PKD.

So, back to my story: with all these potential donors in sight, we decided to go for it, and we proceeded with plans for the double nephrectomy surgery. A few days before the nephrectomy, a colleague, Linda Watson, called to say my transplant coordinator had suggested she call me. I was puzzled about why she was talking to my coordinator. What I did not know was that she had begun donor testing earlier in the fall (my cousin Cindy hadn't started yet). She told me that she knew how disappointed I had been when we found out that neither Mike nor Laurie could be a donor, so she didn't want to risk disappointing me again if things fell through. She then told me that although she had some more testing to do, the team felt confident that all would work out. What a gift and unbelievable sacrifice that she was willing to make for me! What a relief for my family and me with my upcoming surgery to know there was a kidney donor identified.

The double nephrectomy took place right after Thanksgiving, so I was able to enjoy my time with my family a few days beforehand. One very helpful part of the surgical preparation was that I was given pain medication right before the surgery, which is believed to help with pain control both during surgery and afterward. Compared with other surgeries I have had—a hysterectomy, knee surgery—I thought my pain management was much better for the nephrectomy. My scar runs from right above my pubic area to just above my belly button, so it's a whopper, but that enabled the surgeon to take out both kidneys at once without having to make cuts on each side.

The surgery went well and I progressed fairly rapidly, and it helped that I was in generally good health beforehand, other than the UTIs. The biggest part to overcome was the pain from having so much cut out of me. My kidneys by then weighed approximately five pounds each (normal is about three to six ounces!), so if you can imagine having a five-pound bag of sugar on each side of your abdomen and then having them cut away—it was pretty rough. In fact, because I looked as if I was seven to eight months pregnant before the surgery, everywhere I went people asked when my baby was due. I learned that if I told the truth and said I had kidney disease, people would get embarrassed and be really uncomfortable. So if they were strangers and I was unlikely to see them again, I just smiled and said the baby was due in a couple of months. A few years later, when I found a picture of me in a bathing suit, I realized the picture must have been taken right before the nephrectomy. Seeing how big I was, it was no wonder people thought I was at least eight months pregnant!

This memory brings up the whole idea of body image, and if you too have PKD, you know where I'm going with this. For someone who was always slim—my sisters called me Olive Oyl (Popeye's girlfriend) until I was out of high school—this size issue was a big one for me. During my pregnancy with my second child and through the growth hormones supporting the growth of the fetus that kicked in with him (and helped feed my cysts), I went from having a little pooch that came with my daughter's birth to looking perpetually pregnant. I had always wondered why my mom, despite being slim, always had a little tummy pooch, and of course it was her PKD kidneys. My two sisters with PKD were lucky to have had their children in their twenties before the PKD onset (which typically appears in your thirties) and so did not have to deal with growth hormones multiplying the number and size of their cysts. My children were born when I was thirty-eight and forty-two—after the PKD onset. The joys of being an older mother are many, but having a huge belly is not one of them. After the surgery, the sad news was that although my kidneys were gone, my cyst-filled liver (it's polycystic too) began to fill up the empty space. So, I now only look about three to four months pregnant, and still, even at sixty-nine occasionally get asked when my baby is due! I guess I should be flattered.

Because a person can function for only about two to six weeks without a kidney, the day after the surgery an access port was put in my neck for the start of dialysis. I can't remember exactly, but dialysis must have started that day or the next. I don't remember much about dialysis at the hospital because I was still on a fair amount of pain medication and was mostly sleeping and recovering. I will add that the care I received was wonderful and very personalized to my needs. I felt very blessed to have such highly skilled and warm professionals caring for me.

After leaving the hospital, I began to have routine dialysis three times a week at a center near my home. The staff (with only a few exceptions) were highly competent, caring people who were very professional in their interactions with me. The time commitment for the patient is pretty big in that you are usually on the machine for three and a half hours, plus fifteen minutes to get you set up and fifteen minutes to unhook you. They have TV monitors at each station in case you want to watch. I would usually bring a book or magazine to read, plus crossword puzzles and my laptop. Once I went back to work, I usually spent the first two hours working and the last hour reading for pleasure (my reward).

The hardest parts of dialysis for me were the dietary restrictions and guidelines—low salt, potassium, and phosphorus; lots of protein—and watching much more carefully what I ate. The daily fluid restrictions of 32 ounces did not bother me as much, because I was never a big drinker and usually only drank liquids with meals. As Carol mentioned, each session before and after you have dialysis, they weigh you to determine your "dry weight," and then through a formula created for you, they determine how much fluid they should draw off each time. If they draw off too much, you can start cramping. Over time, they got better at the calculations and I had less cramping.

Another issue for me, having borderline hypoglycemia (low blood sugar), was that the rules of the dialysis center at that time did not allow eating during dialysis. I would usually eat a bunch of snacks before going (a hard-boiled egg, cheese and crackers, or other protein), but still I would have very low blood sugar when I came out and would be feeling weak and sometimes nauseous. Another result of my low blood sugar was that if it went too low during dialysis, then I would have little crashes, where I would feel very faint and sick to my stomach. Over time, I began to recognize the early symptoms of low blood sugar and could warn them to slow down my dialysis. Eventually I even talked the staff into letting me nibble on some crackers and cheese during dialysis, and things got much better. I think most dialysis centers now allow their patients to snack during the sessions.

In the beginning, scheduling the sessions wasn't an issue because in the first four to six weeks I wasn't yet back at work so I had much more flexibility. For this period I was happy to take the least popular shift, the middle of the day, but as I neared going back to work I asked and was able to move to the last shift of the day, 3 to 7 p.m. That way I could get in a fair workday and then go to dialysis. Because my boss was flexible and knew that I was working part of the time during dialysis, I didn't have to take any sick leave or time off during those months. I was also fortunate that I did not need to have a fistula surgically placed in my arm or elsewhere, because my doctors hoped I would only be on dialysis a short time given that I now had a potential donor. Instead they used the catheters in my neck, which made my dialysis process relatively painless. The one drawback to neck access is the risk of infection. Compared to others, though, my access story was an easy one.

I felt so good about the tender dialysis care I received that after it was completed, I had a platter of sandwiches delivered to the staff one day for lunch to thank them. My note said, "You guys are the best and I and my family are grateful for your outstanding care, and for caring so deeply about your patients." Although dialysis was time consuming and not always pleasant, during that time I often reminded myself of the luxury I had three times a week to be in a relatively quiet setting where I could read or relax. Yes, I realize I only had to do it for four months and knew it would be temporary, and I didn't have the years on end to deal with. But some of handling dialysis, I think, is a state of mind about framing your experience into something more positive and trying to make the best of the circumstances (yes, I know that's easy for me to say).

My recovery went well and I made excellent progress in reducing the pain medication, gradually increasing the time I spent walking around the house. Overall, I was feeling very fortunate. Then, because I probably failed to listen to the warnings about overdoing it, I had a setback. One day, after carrying a small stack of three or four towels upstairs, I suddenly felt a tearing sensation down my side. I slid to the floor in agony. My side felt as if someone had taken a knife and sliced me from above my ribs way down toward my hip. When I reached my surgeon, he seemed to feel that I had probably pulled out a few stitches and reminded me of the large amount of cutting they had done to take out both of my huge kidneys. Needless to say, I took a few steps back in my recovery, returned to the pain meds, and drastically reduced my activity level. Once I began to feel better, I slowly returned to more activity and was able to again shed the pain meds. If you go through surgery like this, be smarter than I was and work harder at trying not to do too much too soon. It's not worth the risk of a setback.

After being on sick leave for approximately six weeks, I began to gradually return to work. I had been doing some work at home and had been able to return to driving. The first few days, I typically stayed a half-day and then gradually increased to full-time. Those first days, I went home and took a nap, but as I gradually gained back my stamina I was able to work a full day.

It was soon after I had returned to work that Linda finally finished her testing and was approved to be my donor. When she came to my office to tell me, I couldn't believe the news, and of course we were both in tears. When I asked Linda when she wanted to do the transplant, I thought that as a professor like me she would likely want to do it in the summer, when neither of us had teaching responsibilities. Instead she said, "Let's do it as soon as we can, because now that I have my courage up, I don't want to wait any longer." Linda knew I had to wait until at least March to recover from the double nephrectomy, so I was astonished when she suggested we do the transplant during spring break!

Getting Ready for the Transplant

As my recovery continued from my nephrectomy and with my dialysis, my main job was to keep myself healthy until the transplant in March. I did everything I was told: took my medications on time, kept to my strict dialysis diet, stayed away from large groups of people, and started getting a little more exercise in anticipation of being laid up again. As I relate in Part Three, I didn't attend nearly enough to my family's emotional needs at the time, but I did think about their meal and carpooling needs. I set up a website where friends could sign up to help. As the days got closer, we all got excited and a bit anxious. The day of the surgery, Linda and I both checked into the hospital and were able to see each other for a few emotional minutes before she was taken into surgery. They took Linda first to make sure all was well before they took me. The surgery was fairly short compared with the nephrectomy, so I was in recovery pretty soon.

After the surgery, the surgeon reported that once the team had inserted and connected my new kidney, it "pinked right up" and they knew it was going to be a success—such comforting news. Visitors I had at that time all remarked on how much pinker my skin was and how much my coloring had improved. For those of you anticipating a transplant, this surgery was the easy part, honestly. The next day I was sitting up in bed reading a magazine when Linda came down from her room to see me (I was advised not to leave my room because of the risk of infection). Of course, I was pleased to see her but felt awful for her as she looked and probably felt much worse than I did. The nurse told me that it is common for the donor to feel worse initially, but she also said that Linda would leave the hospital sooner than me, recover faster, and get back to work sooner, and she was right on all three counts. Once Linda's doctors got her pain management under control, she began to recover more comfortably. Her sweet husband took off that week and the next to take care of her, and I think after that she went back to work at least part-time. Amazing!

In addition to the wonderful gift of life, Linda had also given me a small bracelet that a friend of hers had made for each of us, with varied stones for different kinds of health: four stones for good kidney health, four for good post-operative healing, and four for general good health. We both wore them right up to surgery, and afterward as soon as they allowed us to put them back on. Several times during our hospital stay, when nurses came in to check on me and noticed my bracelet, they'd say, "There's a woman down the hall with a bracelet just like yours," and I would proudly say, "I know: that's my donor, and she gave me this bracelet to match hers!"

One of the restrictions for transplant recipients to remember is that you can't have any flowers around you for weeks, because of the risk of infection from the soil. Be sure to tell family and friends not to waste their money unless they just want to reward the great nursing staff, who were generally the recipients of my flowers.

I couldn't finish this chapter without talking about the tremendous responsibility I felt for taking care of this precious gift of Linda's kidney. In the days after the transplant, the doctors and nurses gave me plenty of reading material—and I read every word—about my new kidney, its care, and what I could and couldn't do over the next weeks, months, years, and for my lifetime. One day after reading some of the literature, I was suddenly overcome with the heavy feeling of responsibility in needing to take care of Linda's kidney. To think that this person had given me one of her organs—what if I blew it somehow and wasn't responsible enough to give it the care it needed? I don't know why I hadn't previously thought of that aspect of getting a kidney, but it seemed almost crushing at the time and stayed with me throughout the next few days. I talked it over with the surgeon and my nephrologist, and they each reminded me of my usual conscientiousness in my medical care and expressed their confidence that I would do fine. And eventually my practical and optimistic side began to take over, and I realized that it was unlikely that I was going to fall off the rails just because I had a new kidney—I figured it would just make me more relentless about taking care of my, and its, health. Taking a bunch of pills throughout the day and having frequent checkups would be part of my normal routine, but what a small price to pay for a rich and full life.

I couldn't finish this chapter without also talking about my debt to Linda. Of course, the joys of having a new kidney have no bounds, and to feel good again was such a blessing. Not only did I feel better almost instantly, but the thought of no more dialysis or strict dietary restrictions was wonderful. The relief to myself and my family was also such a big boost, and especially to know that I could finally get on to the next part of my life without being so constrained. My debt to Linda and how to thank her lurked in the back of my mind for some time after the transplant. How do you thank someone who has given a part of herself in such a selfless way? The first thing my husband and I did was to ask her husband about ideas for a gift, and knowing what a gardener she was, we wondered about some kind of tree or shrub. Her husband said that ever since they had first moved to Redbud Lane, they had always talked about getting a redbud tree. So that's what we got: a nice, mature redbud. When we went over to plant it in Linda's front yard, it was wonderful to see her face at the sight of their new tree! It also seemed fitting that she gave a life to me and got one in return, although only a green one.

Despite the tree, I was still left with a sense of not knowing how to thank Linda enough. She helped me gain a sense of peace with a card she sent me after the transplant. On the front of the card was a picture of a lovely flying swan and the words "All that the human experience is about is the journey to wholeness." On the inside, Linda had written, "You have said, 'You will never be able to thank me.' But I think the experience has been equally powerful in a positive way for me. Hopefully, my kidney will contribute to your physical well-being for years to come. Taking this step to give it contributes to me in a more spiritual journey toward wholeness." Reading those powerful words was the first time that I realized that the experience had contributed to her life too, so it eased my burden of insufficient thanks.

In closing, if you or someone you love is considering a kidney transplant, I can't say enough about taking the leap if you can. The renewed health I have had over these last sixteen years has been such a gift that I can't imagine my life without this astounding treasure.

CHAPTER 11

Lessons Learned: Our Do's and Don'ts

After reading our personal stories, you know that we both acquired a lot of useful information about donation and transplant the hard way. We want to share some of those tips here.

Mostly Medical Matters

CAROL

1. Be patient, and be prepared for a potentially months-long donor evaluation process.

2. Ask lots of questions and take notes. Review your notes at home, and if anything is unclear, ask again. Learn as much as you can.

3. Take one step at a time, and don't worry about reaching a point of no return in your decision to donate. Knowing I could always change my mind—up to the moment of the surgery—gave me the confidence to keep going.

4. If you're a wimp like me, don't be embarrassed to share your nervousness with the donor coordinator. He or she can keep that in mind and offer helpful tips (like using lidocaine before blood draws) and perhaps recommend another professional on the team for you to talk to.

5. In general, don't feel that you can't betray any hesitation or fear. The transplant team and the nursing staff are well aware that this is a big step. I found that they weren't just accommodating, but treated me with understanding and admiration.

6. Stay in shape: get plenty of exercise, and eat well. Staying healthy is important both for your sake and your recipient's.

7. If you feel as well as I did after the surgery, don't be tempted to overdo it. Remember not to lift heavy objects and to rest as much as you need. Enjoy a guilt-free nap in the afternoon!

8. Once you're no longer under the surgeon's care, tell your providers that you should avoid taking NSAIDs whenever there is a viable alternative. With just one kidney, it's best to stay away from drugs that are known to be damaging to kidneys.

9. Have your creatinine and blood pressure checked every year—it's the only lab work that needs to be monitored specifically for a living donor. If your creatinine is fine and all is well, don't be concerned about a lower-than-normal GFR—that's typical for a healthy person with one kidney.

10. Do not be shy about telling people you are a living donor. Most people react with awe and disbelief, particularly if it's just weeks after the transplant, and they generally imagine a far more debilitating post-op period. You never know—you just might inspire others to consider donating a kidney themselves.

BETSY

1. Don't learn about your kidney function the hard way, as I did. Everyone with kidney disease needs to be as well informed as possible and understand the potential ramifications regarding both short- and long-term outcomes. Always know your "numbers," and use them to actively help your doctor plan the next steps in your healthcare, rather than the other way around.

2. It may be helpful to talk to all your providers about your own preferences for being informed about medical information and about their style of communicating with you, the patient. Now as I meet new doctors, I find this kind of conversation helpful to have at the very beginning so there is no doubt about my role in making decisions about my own healthcare.

3. If you have PKD, you may need to do some work with yourself or a professional about your body image and how to keep your head on straight

about what's important, and recognize it's not worth worrying about how your body looks to others.

4. Identify all the options for dialysis and help in the decision making with your medical team about which type is the best for you. Also, remember that some people do multiple types of dialysis serially, so once a decision is made it doesn't have to be permanent.

5. If you're on dialysis, think about getting yourself on the transplant list and off dialysis. It will likely lengthen your life and will most certainly improve your health now and for the future.

6. Keep in mind the insurance ramifications of the transplant. Talk with the transplant social worker to identify what is and is not covered.

7. If you need a transplant, don't be shy about telling your story and your need for a donated kidney, and encouraging others to do the same. Think of all possible avenues: family, work, school, faith community, and volunteer organizations, because you never know where a kidney may come from.

8. If you have a donor who isn't a good match for you, ask your transplant team about paired donation or a donor-chain possibility. Many transplant centers now have mechanisms for handling cases in which a potential donor who isn't a match for you may be a match for another person in a "swap" or chain.

9. If you're waiting for or getting ready for a transplant, read all you can about what to expect.

10. My sister Barbara, who went through a few false alarms before receiving a kidney from a deceased donor, had this advice: always be prepared to be disappointed on the first call, or even subsequent ones, when you go in for testing for a possible kidney. Eventually there will be one for you too!

Feelings, Family, and Friends

1. *Accept* all offers of help. People don't offer if they don't mean it (and if they really don't mean it, that'll teach them not to make empty offers!).

2. *Ask* for help when you or your family needs it. If you don't feel comfortable doing it yourself, ask a friend to set up a site, listserv, meal delivery list, etc. Remember, your friends and family want to help in a big way. They just don't always know how or when. So tell them!

3. Be sure, too, to take care of yourself and let others know what you need emotionally.

4. Take advantage of built-in mechanisms for support, such as having a realtor sell your house, using care providers, or using flextime at work.

5. Keep your family's and friends' emotional well-being in mind too, as you move through your journey for a transplant.

6. Think of your spouse's or partner's perspective. Even though an adult, he or she has needs and concerns that may be separate or opposite from yours.

7. Be sure to tell your child's teachers (and perhaps coaches and counselors) about your family situation so they can be alert to any problems.

8. If you have teenagers, be ever more watchful, because they are typically struggling with their own hard times and may be less likely to open up about their feelings.

9. Do what you can to find little ways to make the patient smile, laugh (even better), or enjoy something to help get through dialysis or difficult times in general.

10. Don't hesitate, when it's important, to contact providers at home if they have offered that option—nor to ask for it, if they haven't.

11. Don't feel that you have to make an important judgment call alone—for example, see #10.

12. In awkward social situations, such as when someone you haven't seen in a long time says "So how have you been?" practice saying "We've been dealing with some health issues." If need be, add "that I'd rather not go into right now."

13. Laugh as much as possible. Look for the humor in every situation. If you can't find any, try watching laugh-out-loud movies or TV episodes.

14. Remember that there is no shame in needing to raise funds for a transplant or living donation.

15. Take comfort in good news along the way, but don't take the news for granted or get ahead of yourself—anything could delay or derail donor testing, surgery scheduling, or financing.

16. Seek professional help to guide you and your family if you feel that would be useful to open up strong channels of communication.

Part Three:
Family Dynamics

*The decision to donate your kidney or to undergo
a transplant, like many major health decisions, affects the
whole family. How we communicate with loved ones during
these stressful times can help ease—or add—tension.*

CHAPTER 12

Helping Manage
the Emotional Process

by Kathleen Fitzgerald

Kathleen Fitzgerald is a Licensed Professional Counselor, teacher, and trainer in Chapel Hill, North Carolina.

LIVING WITH ANY CHRONIC ILLNESS is difficult and painful physically, emotionally, relationally, and mentally. End-stage renal disease (ESRD) is tough on families. It often strikes when people are in the prime of their lives. They have dreams, jobs, financial responsibilities, families, and hopes, and then they are sick, facing long and painful physical issues and treatments, and, for some, eventually the need for a kidney.

Families face the illness, and all of its issues too, because chronic illness affects everyone in the family. I have had the opportunity to work with a number of families dealing with ESRD and have seen how family members respond to the illness, each in his or her own unique way. Different families handle issues in different ways and at a different pace. Some families accept the illness and work together, handling the complexities with ease. Usually these families communicate well, are empathic, listen to one another, and learn new skills together.

Other families struggle. Family members are often scared. Fear is not always demonstrated gracefully or dealt with directly; and if others dismiss or minimize it, all too frequently fear manifests as angry behavior. Even with the best of intentions, rigid, limiting, dismissive, and hurtful patterns of communication and engagement can result. Some family members feel the need for self-protection as well as to protect others. All too often families find themselves in the pitfalls of disconnection. Instead of bonding together, when the going gets tough, members disengage and grow more distant. The result is a family whose members love one another but lose touch, even if they are living under the same roof.

In a typical parental response, parents often think they should know exactly what to say so no one gets upset. It is helpful for adults to recognize their need to fix things, but sometimes there *is* no solution or *need* to fix, and parents benefit from knowing that they do not need to have all the answers. Sometimes listening and understanding are what's needed.

Illnesses take center stage. Families frequently err in making everything about the illness. But relationships have a way of making themselves visible. Unfortunately, the illness usurps energy, and the relationships then get wrapped around the illness. Yet families are vitally essential to all of us, especially when there is an illness.

How Different Families Handle Complex Emotions

We are born into families, and it is within the family structure that we learn how to interact with and attach to others. Everyone is born with the ability to recognize and respond accordingly to the eight primary emotions: joy, curiosity or interest, sadness, anger, fear, shock, doubt, and shame or guilt. The family unit teaches us which emotions are acceptable and how to respond to thoughts, feelings, and behaviors, as well as conflict and challenges. Given that this is done without direct instruction, how to deal with hard emotions is learned unconsciously.

When family members bravely share their feelings, they become closer. But some people avoid their feelings and become numb when vulnerable. In general, people who love each other do not know how to talk about complicated subjects, so they develop all kinds of behaviors to avoid awkwardness.

ESRD causes stress, and stress makes people feel vulnerable. Children are particularly vulnerable. Some parents, instead of reacting by needing to resolve the situation, alternatively overprotect their children. They tell them that all will be fine and that they have nothing to worry about. But the children are already worried and now they do not know what to do with their worries—they quickly learn they cannot tell their parents about these concerns. Or the parents give them far too many medical facts, few of which children or even teens truly understand or need to know. Again, the children are overwhelmed.

Let's consider how a few different families have dealt with the emotional complexities of ESRD and the need for a transplant.

When Kids Don't Express Their Fears

One family I worked with had a fifteen-year-old daughter, Susan, who had attention deficit hyperactivity disorder (ADHD) and learning disabilities. Her mom had kidney disease. Susan did not walk—she flew, talking nonstop, hands waving in the air, often pretending to be an Elf from Middle Earth. She was part of a group for teens with ADHD. For more than a year, this group met weekly. During that year, Susan's mother grew quite ill from her disease and elected to have her kidneys removed in preparation for a future kidney transplant.

The week of the surgery, at the teen group, Susan lay under the snack table, and, using an entire roll of duct tape, taped the legs together, tears dripping down her face for the full two-hour group session. She wanted to talk about how upset she was with her parents. She said they kept their conversations regarding what was happening to her mother to just the facts: what, where, when. Susan wanted to let them know how frightened and upset she was. She wanted to ask, "Is mom going to die?" Her parents often said, "Oh, don't worry; everything will be fine," or "We are not going to talk about sad things." As time went on, Susan's anxiety grew, and she started thinking about hurting herself.

After coming to see me, Susan's family began to hold family meetings with me. Each person in the family had five to ten minutes to talk about his or her feelings and thoughts. The goal was for them to listen to one another. No one was to give advice! No one was to try to fix the others' feelings by telling them not to worry, what to do, or to calm down. This was very hard for Susan's mother, her brother would become agitated and yell at people to stop talking, and her father would sit in despair because he hated conflict.

With assistance, Susan's parents gradually learned to listen and not give advice. I suggested they look at each other to keep each other calm. Susan also learned many strategies for keeping herself calm so she could listen to others. Often, she had to sit on her hands. As Susan realized that her parents were listening while she talked, she began to feel calmer. As time went on, her thoughts of hurting herself became less intense and less frequent.

When Partners Distance Themselves

Partners face struggles also. The partner who is sick often worries about being a burden or abandoned. The healthy partner often feels burdened by the illness, financial concerns, and caregiving. Partners who share their concerns become closer and feel valued and understood as they face the illness together. However, many partners are afraid to share their feelings. As a result, a distance grows between them, which makes both feel more lonely. People engage in a variety of behaviors to distance themselves from pain. Isolation comes in many forms; some adults drink or overwork. Some distance their loved ones with their anger, by yelling, or by criticizing themselves or others.

Vivian was a fierce, smart, energetic sprinter who earned a law degree. A few years after joining a local firm she was made a partner. She had plans for her life and let nothing interfere. She fell in love with a man in law school, a kind, smart, soft-spoken man, and they married after graduation. They wanted to work hard, see the world, have a child. Several years after they married, her husband began to feel weak, and before he was forty, he was diagnosed with polycystic kidney disease. Within a few years he was having daily dialysis at home and was on the transplant list. Vivian decided to fix the problem. She would give her husband a kidney. As she began the process, her law partners were anxious: what if she didn't survive? The livelihood of the firm depended on her strong work. Eventually they asked her to leave. No worries: Vivian opened her own firm. She travelled more, worked longer hours, and left a sick husband—and now their small child—at home.

Tension began to build between Vivian and her husband. His illness caused him a great deal of pain, and physical intimacy became impossible. Even a hug was too painful. Vivian learned that she could not be his donor. At the same time, his health declined rapidly. Regularly he was taken to the hospital, often needing a medical procedure that temporarily made him inactive on the wait lists. Vivian's panic and anger grew.

She knew how to be successful and fix things; she did not know how to tolerate an unfixable situation. An emotional chasm developed between Vivian and her husband. She wondered if there was any point in staying in the marriage. Both felt despair and depression but handled it differently. Vivian got busy: she took more business trips and made more money; she considered having an affair—it had been years since she had been hugged. Her husband became more withdrawn.

They sought help for their marriage. They were stuck in a cycle, but with some help they began to see their pattern of distancing from each other. As their physical intimacy stopped, so had the emotional intimacy. It had been years since he had told Vivian he loved her. Now the couple began to have dates. He was in too much pain for a hug, but he could hold her hand and tell Vivian he loved her. Vivian now felt much more connected to him and remembered how much she loved him. She acknowledged that her frantic working helped her deal with her pent-up anxiety about what was happening to her husband and their marriage.

Together they began to figure out how Vivian could harness her energy in a different way. She joined a running group, and as a family they went together. Her husband would pick up dinner for them to share at the end of the workout. They began to laugh together. When Vivian ran a 5K, her husband met her at the finish line and held her hand and kissed her cheek. He wanted to wrap his arms around her, but he was still in too much pain. By then Vivian had learned to accept his limitations, and the couple found togetherness in other ways.

When Teens Change Their Behavior

Adults may feel they have little control over a seemingly unfixable situation, but children and teens facing chronic family stress have even less control and show their stress by their behavior. Children often become clingy, and demanding. They talk too much or throw tantrums, whining until adults give in to their demands. Some have trouble eating and sleeping. Similarly, teens show their emotional struggles behaviorally. Some find focusing and attending hard and begin to do poorly in school. Others skip classes, and find themselves getting into trouble with drugs or relationships. Often teens withdraw from their families and stop talking to them or become combative, arguing often about family rules such as routine curfews. The teens attempt to avoid talking about things they do not know how to talk about, and this can result in their engaging in behaviors that make their parents mad and worried. Regularly fights erupt, and the parents see their teen's behavior as "bad" instead of related to the family's troubles with discussing difficult topics.

Seth began to have panic attacks as a young teen. He had an awful feeling that someone was going to drain his blood. Sleeping became impossible. Nights were full of vivid nightmares of vampires, long fangs piercing his side, near where his kidneys lodge. Seth's dad had been diagnosed with chronic kidney disease and needed a kidney transplant. Seth hated inviting friends over. Often the dinner conversation after a visit from a friend went like this:

"So, your friend is nice."

Seth would stare and not speak, already dreading the inevitable questions.

"What's his family like? Are they healthy? Have you told them about your father? A nice family would consider donating a kidney."

Seth felt rage inside of him, and he believed he was not allowed to express his true feelings; instead, he exhaled very loudly, clenching his fists under the table.

"I'm tired of your selfishness, Seth. Are you a family member or not?" his mother responded sternly.

Seth began to skip school. He could not sleep and felt physically sick. One day after his mother drove him to school, Seth crept off to a friend's car where he slept. The truancy officer found him and contacted his parents, noting that he had missed ten classes over the past few weeks.

Seth's parents were very angry. Luckily, they came for counseling and were taught to listen and validate (acknowledge and accept) one another's thoughts and feelings. Seth told them he couldn't sleep because he was angry at them for looking at his friends as potential donors. At first his parents said things like, "Don't blame this on us; you're the one skipping classes." The defensive arguments continued to keep them all from understanding each other, connecting, and calming down.

With help, the parents gradually began to listen without interrupting, giving advice, or minimizing how upset Seth was. They began to see how they had responded belligerently to Seth's feelings. Slowly, they learned to take a moment, settle their own feelings, and show concern about his.

When Seth told them about his nightmares, his parents began to see that his behaviors were motivated by his feelings. He was scared. They learned to acknowledge those emotions and respond thoughtfully, saying things like, "You're scared because Dad is so sick, and you're afraid we'll hurt your friends. Well, we wish you weren't skipping classes, but your behavior makes sense." Seth looked at them in disbelief.

It took several weeks, but slowly his parents learned to validate his feelings and sit with their feelings. Slowly the family members began to talk. And gradually, Seth began to sleep well at night and stopped skipping classes.

Doing What's Hardest

Clearly, it is vital for people to do the one thing they are spending a great deal of energy avoiding: talking about things, *especially* scary ones. Talking honestly and openly is hard and sometimes seems against people's better judgment, but it is the key to feeling understood and valued, which brings people together. They feel connected and calmer even when their loved ones are sick.

Reaching this goal takes some effort. Family members need to make time to sit together and talk, listening without interrupting and encouraging the sharing of feelings. Adults need to give appropriate amounts of information—not overload—and be sure to ask about or listen to fears. Parents need to know they have limits and are doing the best they can. Resting together, playing games, and laughing are important. Often families can get back to being happy and having fun together once the emotions are recognized and soothed. In short, people should act as if they matter to each other, and remember how much they love each other.

It is essential for every person in the family to talk about their own concerns, fears, and worries. As I mentioned earlier, many parents try to protect the children by not talking about scary things, but teens and children know something is going on, and often what they imagine is *worse* than reality. Knowing what to say and how to encourage conversation is valuable. It is also important for parents to have reasonable expectations of themselves and their children. The same is true for partners. Finally, adults and children both need to accept that they don't have to fix every situation. Truthfully, they couldn't if they tried.

Interestingly, often behaviors that become problematic were a solution at one point. For example, if a child learns that he or she is not supposed to act frightened when a parent is sick, the child will be numb. Many parents mistakenly view a child's quiet behavior as a relief; they may think the child is just fine and has no worries. In turn, the child learns not to seek out a parent even when the child wants and needs to. The child may engage in different numbing and distracting behaviors such as video gaming; a teen may try drugs, and an adult, like my client Vivian, may disappear into overwork.

Validation

One of the most important things family members can do is *validate* one another's thoughts and feelings. A listener does not have to agree with or like what she hears. Validation encompasses and surpasses empathy. It means hearing and recognizing the feelings, and acknowledging the truth in what is said. Validation has at least three important components:

1. Truly listening, and acknowledging the other person. Listen to understand the other person. Face the other person. Give your whole presence to the other person, listening with interest and curiosity. Do not think about how to respond.

2. Naming the feeling and the thought of the other person. For example, when Susan was gyrating around the house, her parents learned to sit her down and say, "I see your body moving everywhere. I think you have something on your mind."

3. Letting the other person know that what he or she is feeling and thinking makes sense. After Susan began to trust that her parents cared about her experiences, she would tell them what was happening. Her parents responded by saying, "Well, that makes sense."

Emotions are part of each human interaction. We see behaviors, not thoughts and beliefs. We don't see or understand the emotion that underlies and causes the behavior. It is helpful for families to become more knowledgeable about emotions and the complex set of behaviors that make up an emotional interaction.

First, there is a *trigger*. Emotions come from somewhere. They are triggered internally or, often, externally. Someone says or does something, and a reaction is set off. For Susan, as soon as her parents told her not to worry, she was overwhelmed by emotions.

There is an *interpretation*. People give meaning to the act. Susan thought she did not matter. Being told not to worry when she was very worried meant her feelings were not important.

There is also an *internal body experience*. These reactions are involuntary. People will experience their emotions in their body. They may feel some of the following: tightness in muscles, flush in their chest or face, racing in their heart, dryness in the mouth, shakiness in their limbs, and so on. Some people cannot tolerate what they are feeling.

Susan's father was very uneasy with difficult emotions, and he periodically had to leave the room for the first few family sessions. Slowly, he began to understand that the uncomfortable feelings in his body were his emotions. As time went on, he was able to stay in the therapy session with his family. The other family members were taught to let him know that they understood he was overwhelmed and that it was okay for him to leave until he was calm enough to return.

Emotional reactions also have *voluntary physical reactions*. People may furrow their brow, point their finger, make a fist, smile, stare at someone, kick something, or make a face.

There are *action urges*. People will think of all the different things they could say or do. They then pick things to say or do, and the people they are talking to have their own reactions. This all happens very quickly, often in a matter of seconds, which makes people think that emotions come out of nowhere, and that there is nothing that can be done about them or that they are not responsible for their behaviors. However, learning to slow things down, and teaching people to sense what happens to them, allows them to see the choices they are making and to make new and different choices. This is hard work, and people benefit from support so they can see their behaviors and make changes.

Families benefit from learning about emotional reactions and taking some time to understand each person's reactions. These reactions need to be observed and described in kind, nonjudgmental ways. For many people, learning about their own reactions takes a great deal of time and care.

Mindfulness

Many families benefit from practicing mindfulness together. Mindfulness allows people to develop the skills they need so they can see and feel their reactions. They learn more about their own internal processes and how they think and manage their own emotions. People slow down their reactions so they can see the choices they make. Mindfulness helps families change old ways of interacting and develop new patterns.

Regularly, families who confront ESRD will tell me that a fight among them "just happened." It literally came out of nowhere, they say. And yet, when I sit with the family and slowly go through the story, asking when they began to yell, or curse, or criticize, it is clear that there was a trigger, and signs. If people learn to see their own behaviors and take a second to breathe and attend to what is happening, often a conflict can be dealt with differently, and people will feel more supported and understood. Developing skills in mindfulness is often a helpful first step.

Mindfulness encompasses the simple practice of sitting quietly for five or so minutes. Beforehand, family members choose a mindfulness practice, such as noticing sounds or scanning their body. It is predictable that their minds will wander. The goal is to notice where the mind went and bring it back to the chosen focus. What other thoughts, emotions, and body sensations came into the mind during mindfulness? In addition, the person notices judgmental thinking. Everyone has likes, dislikes, preferences, and thoughts. The important thing is to notice when thoughts become harsh and critical. Again, as family members sit in mindfulness, they notice their judgments.

They do not focus on them; they simply register the judgment, let it go, and bring themselves back to focus.

The practice of mindfulness also helps people understand where their minds go. They become fully aware of their thoughts, emotions, body sensations, and judgments. These experiences, if not understood, can become triggers for difficult interactions. Mindfulness lets people see what they are experiencing, and find the deep, calm place inside of them that is able to observe and stay calm. This part of the person can make choices and not be reactive.

It is helpful for a family to practice mindfulness together a few times a week. Once the five minutes are up, family members share their experiences. Some will be able to focus and feel calm right away. Others will have trouble because their brain goes all over. Still others will feel bored. Being able to share experiences in an accepting and nonjudgmental environment helps families feel closer.

In mindfulness, there are no mistakes. Whatever happens is what happens. As families practice mindfulness, they become better at attending to their thoughts, emotions, and sensations. Then, when they are having tough moments with one another, they are better able to take a moment, make choices, and avoid a conflict.

ESRD, like any chronic illness, is tough on families. Happily, there are many skills families can learn that enhance their relationships and support them as they encounter myriad stressors associated with the disease. One skill is mindfulness. It is simple and yet takes time, attention, and focus. It is worth the effort. Families facing living donation or transplant also benefit from validating each other: listening with true curiosity, ready to find out what is going on with their loved ones, and letting them know that their behavior makes sense. Perhaps most of all, families benefit from talking about what is going on: sharing their fears and concerns, and making time to be together.

CHAPTER 13

What One Family's Missteps Taught Them

Betsy's transplant and the varied ways that her family experienced it illustrate some of the difficult emotional issues families contend with in trying times. Here she recalls the painful lessons she learned through the admittedly less-than-graceful way she and her husband handled their own very stressful situation.

I WOULDN'T CALL MYSELF INSENSITIVE, and I think my friends and students consider me a caring person, but I sure blew it in not paying enough attention to my own family before, during, and after my kidney surgeries.

A Word About My Upbringing

The backdrop to this story: I was raised by an engineer father who was fiercely independent and mostly just wanted to get on with business and not be distracted by all the niceties of small talk, not by recognizing and certainly not talking about anyone's feelings. A quick story about my dad exemplifies his own occasional obliviousness to others. One summer, we were readying a friend's boat for a ride. My dad rushed past me and inadvertently knocked me in the water. When I popped up, his first response was to yell at me for getting in *his* way! Clearly, he was upset about what he'd done, but instead of comforting me, he reacted with blame.

My mother too, although thoughtful and giving at times, was also very self-directed and did not always attend to things not on her agenda. Once when I was little and cut my foot, she washed it, put on a Band-Aid, and then rushed off to a meeting. When my dad came home he took me to the doctor, where I had seven stitches and a tetanus shot. I guess you could say my mother was the opposite of an alarmist.

My parents were fine people and loved us very much, but their Depression-era backgrounds instilled in them the philosophy behind many adages of the day: "pull yourself up by the bootstraps" and "if you don't stop crying, I'll give you something to cry about." Throughout most situations, my family has always taken a positive, yet practical view. We look on the bright side, unlike my husband's family, who see disaster around every corner, and even among my family I'm known for having rose-colored corneas.

Given this history, it is no wonder that I approached my transplant with little thought of what my husband and children, or friends, were feeling or thinking. This reflection on my upbringing is not to justify my blitheness in considering my own family and friends during the lead-up to and during my transplant, but just to give a picture of how I was raised and some of the traits I internalized along the way.

Much later, after it was all over, I felt terribly insensitive when I learned that my teenaged daughter, Rachael, had gone into a weekly group she belonged to and said, "Guess what, my mother is going to have a transplant and she might die." Then a couple of weeks later she told the group, "It gets even better, my dad now may be my mom's donor, and they both might die." At the time I didn't know how Rachael was feeling, because first, I failed to ask, and second, I was feeling positive about the whole thing and I guess I figured everyone else was too.

A few weeks earlier, I had told both our kids (Rachael was then fourteen, and Sam was ten) that I needed to have my kidneys taken out and later would need a transplant. Whenever I talked to them about either surgery, I was very upbeat and mentioned my good health and likely speedy recovery, with little attention to any negative possibilities, certainly not death. In contrast to my factual and optimistic approach, when any of these health issues arose, particularly the possibility of a poor outcome, my husband's approach was to quickly change the topic and usually say, "Let's not dwell on anything negative or sad."

And to show you further evidence of my cluelessness, I even sent both kids to school on the days of my two surgeries. Knowing that my husband would be a worried mess, I figured he would have less to deal with if the kids were in school, and they would be distracted by their usual activities. It never occurred to me that they all might be a comfort to one another. Unfortunately, on the day of my transplant, as I later learned, Rachael heard her name on the loudspeaker calling her to the school office. By the time she arrived, she was sobbing and the staff were perplexed that she was so upset—they hadn't yet told her they were concerned about her behavior in a class. Finally, she was able to get out the words: "I thought you were calling to tell me my mother had died!" Clearly, we had not been sensitive enough to think about alerting the school to my surgery or talking with the school counselors in case either of the kids needed extra support. So it's no wonder that the kids found little space to talk about any of their feelings with a mother who was oblivious to their concerns and who only saw a rosy outcome, and a father who didn't want to hear or talk about anything worrisome or scary.

What I Would Do Differently If I Had the Chance

You may have a different situation in terms of whether you have a life partner, children, living parents, in-laws, and close friends that you need to keep in the loop. You also probably have a better sense than I did of who can handle what information and when. If I had been wiser, I think I would have started some of the hard conversations with our kids about what was going to happen a bit sooner, to give them more time to think about it and to ask needed questions. I would also make sure I asked them often about their feelings and to see if they had further questions or concerns. Given that my son is a worrier like my husband, and my daughter is a little more stoic like me, I would also have tried harder to individualize my attention to their needs, especially as to how much we talked about the surgeries. If I had been more cognizant of Sam's need to talk things out at the time of the surgeries, I would have spent more time just listening rather than immediately assuring him and thereby stifling his thoughts and feelings.

Rachael is usually quite expressive, but at the time was fully into adolescence (a scary time anyway and often a time of limited communication with parents), so I think we mistook her quietness for adolescent-hood. I didn't find out until later that she was scared to death for me and didn't want to bring up the subject, and certainly not with her already anxious father. So Rachael just sat on her feelings and simultaneously began to get the worst grades of her academic life, eventually failing two classes. Setting up opportunities for the kids to express themselves could have helped immeasurably.

Now to my husband. Everyone who knows Mike thinks he is a really mellow guy who can easily brush things off his sleeve. But what they don't know is that every day he has his own bundle of anxieties on the inside. As opposed to my way of thinking, which is always that the glass is half full, he is definitely a glass-half-empty kind of guy. For example, when I suggest we go someplace to eat, instead of saying, "Oh, honey, that sounds like a great idea," his first response is usually, "I bet there's already a line and it's going to be crowded." You would have thought that after having lived with him for twenty-one years I would have recognized and anticipated his needs too, but I didn't. I think I was fooled by his calm exterior, although his typical "going into mourning mode" a few days before I went on trips, and certainly when I was going to the hospital, should have given me a clue about how worried he was. By mourning, I mean telling me how much he and the kids will miss me, offering to pick up the dry cleaning, going to the pharmacy for me, or reminding me to be sure to take along my meds. It's his way whenever I travel to help me get ready, but in reality it masks his worry about something happening either to me or to the kids while I'm gone. If I could go back in time, I would have anticipated this worry on his part and both spent more time with him and talked to him more about his feelings and concerns.

What we did do right, after the fact, was get together with two family therapists who often worked as a team and already knew our family. They skillfully spent time with the four of us, walking us through (and drawing up a long wall-chart timeline of) our journey through the whole process. We were all seated opposite the wall where we could easily see the chart. As they had us remember and talk about our journey, they would write up approximate dates in chronological order and the event that was taking place at that time. They started with our first awareness of my need for surgery and our first discussion of it with our kids. At that point and during each additional phase along the way, they had each of us think back to those times and talk about our feelings and thoughts about what was happening—the impending surgery, their dad as a possible donor.

At first the kids talked little about their feelings and more about the facts of the event, such as what was going on at school and home at the time. Fortunately, the therapists were very good at making them feel safe and not pressured, while gently encouraging them to express their real feelings. Gradually the kids began to open up and say more about how afraid they were at various times and how hesitant they were to bring up any worries or fears to either Mike or me. This was how I found out about what Rachael had told her group (that her parents might die) and about being called to the office on the day of the transplant. As you can imagine, it was a very emotional time for all of us and each of us cried at various stages, sometimes at multiple stages. I personally felt so inadequate as a parent (and wife) and couldn't believe how insensitive I had been to all of my family's fears and needs. I know Mike felt badly too that he had not recognized more of what was going on for our kids and had not been able to move beyond his own worries to help address theirs. He also shared with all of us how afraid he was of losing me and how much he worried about what would happen to him and the kids without me. Since I'm the master organizer of the household and our family's activities (doctor visits, school communications, bills, travel plans, meals, Boy and Girl Scout activities, holiday events), I think Mike was terrified of losing not only the love of his life, but also the glue that kept our family together. I can only imagine what terror he endured during the whole process, especially not being able to talk about it.

Needless to say, this process of walking and talking through our journey was one of the best and most therapeutic things that happened to all of us. I was so grateful to the two therapists and how they had led us to much more peace and understanding of the events surrounding the whole process. It was only through these sessions that Mike and I began to realize how few opportunities we had given our kids to share their current feelings (and our own feelings) and to address them when they were most acute. Another benefit of the sessions was that they helped change some of our interaction styles with our kids and each other, and we learned to be more mindful of our own and our kids' feelings and to share them more freely with each other. Sam's way to handle something scary or sad (after a lot of work) is now to process it out loud and just talk about it over and over until he gets more settled about it. Although the repetition at times gets a little tiresome, the best part is that he does make us more aware of his feelings and has found a strategy that works for him. Rachael also has learned to be more open about her feelings with each of us and not hold things in to her own detriment.

If I had it to do over, I would definitely seek the help of one or more professionals early on to guide us periodically through the process, or at the least be sure to provide more opportunities for deep discussion with our kids without one of us brushing off their concerns. It would also have been helpful to read more about handling these kinds of emotional issues with my family and friends, but I wasn't aware (or made aware by the professionals working with us) of this type of printed material. What a shame to not have been able to get some guidance beforehand to help us attend to our children's needs and support them as best we could. This lack of guidance and my own blunders will always be a regret I have about that time in our lives.

One of the things I did do well was accept help before and during the process. One of the best things that I did was to set up a web-based group site. There are many, like Helpinghands.org and CaringBridge.org, that make it easy for friends and relatives to help you. Most have calendars where you can list the dates and times when you need help, such as with meals, rides to doctor's appointments or dialysis treatments, rides for your children to activities, and medication or grocery pickups. (I had used both websites for other people and found them endlessly useful in telling me when and how to help.) My friends and work colleagues helpfully set up a system for driving me to and from dialysis and dubbed it the "Driving Miss Betsy" list.

Three especially helpful meal-related options let people know what dietary restrictions I had (especially important while on dialysis), along with websites for dialysis recipes, and a place where people could list the food they were planning to bring us, so that we didn't get two fettuccini Alfredos in a week. My son so much liked these meals that months later he suggested I have surgery again so we could get more delivered meals! The website also gave us one place to spread the word about my recovery, so we didn't need to email everyone separately and wonder whom we had left out of the loop. That allowed people to check the site for updates and learn about our current needs. Another alternative to keep people in the loop is an email listserv.

So finally, don't be afraid to help others help *you*—they will welcome your guidance (at least that's what my friends and colleagues told me).

CHAPTER 14

A Parent's Crisis,
a Teen's Dilemma

Even when children or teens don't readily express their fears about a parent's looming health problems, they often show their concerns in subtle ways—and sometimes in distressing ones. Here Betsy's daughter, Rachael, candidly recalls her experiences around the transplant and offers advice to both parents and teens facing a similarly traumatic health crisis together.

by Rachael Crais Wagner

MY MOTHER IS THE BACKBONE of our family. She's the spinal cord that brings everyone together. She helps the rest of us navigate through the world and, as I continue to find, she's a huge part of our communication. To our core, she's our rock, the cool head in the storm. When she gets damaged, whether by a cold or something far more serious, it's felt throughout the whole family.

All this is to say that when she went through the story I'm about to tell you—some of which she's already shared in this book—it was terrifying for my teenage self. This strong woman warrior, who conquered every fear I had and still managed to make dinner most nights (Dad, I'm calling you out), got her kidneys removed during my sophomore year in high school.

When she was brought low by this terrible disease, it shook my whole world and my understanding of how the world existed. I had never heard of polycystic kidney disease, or PKD, until she was telling me about her "numbers" and that the doctors might have to remove both of her kidneys. She was so somber and serious that I knew right then this was going to be bigger than my father and she were letting on. My father was talking about donating a kidney to her. And my selfish teenage mind went right to the fear that no one would be around to take care of my little brother and me. I was still going to school by bus, so how would we visit them in the hospital?

With an awful sort of relief on my part, we soon found out that my dad's donating was not an option. To my mother's fury and my father's remorse, his previous melanoma disqualified him all along, despite his early disclosure. You see, he got almost through the donor testing when they told him, and disappointment was all he got for his time. All I remember was the sadness on his face when he told us he couldn't be the match. I know it hurts him to this day that he couldn't help my mom in her hour of need.

Sometimes when I asked about the initial diagnosis or other issues about the transplant process, my mom didn't always seem to know the answers. I think in some ways her lack of initial knowledge and understanding about the predicament made me even more worried back then. She's not a medical doctor, and I shouldn't have expected her to know the ins and outs of everything while she was just learning it herself, but I did. This woman, who knows everything, doesn't know about this?

High school is already hard. Now imagine going through it while wondering if your mom is dying. I had so many questions: Will she be plugged into machines the rest of her life? How long does dialysis work? Does it stop working? When do people show signs? Are these things—the cysts—growing in me too? Am I next? After learning that I had a 50–50 chance of inheriting PKD, I couldn't stop these morbid thoughts.

I wrote two poems while in high school about my newfound relationship with PKD that I think will help you understand my headspace at the time. The first I showed to my mom, and the other I kept for myself:

JUST A STUPID KIDNEY

by Rachael Crais Wagner

Just a stupid kidney.

One small insignificant organ.

You know, the one that cleans the blood.

The one it's hard to survive without.

The one my Mom needs.

Dialysis three times a week, Monday, Wednesday and Thursday.

Mom looks like she's pregnant, but I know better.

People often ask her "When is it due?"

It is hard to answer, "There is no baby. I have a kidney disease."

It hasn't happened yet.

She still has one working.

But I know there's not much time left.

It's also hereditary; I probably have it too.

PKD stands for Polycystic Kidney Disease

Or for Pity Kindly Declined

Or perhaps People Keep Dying.

Just a stupid kidney.

A stupid, stupid kidney.

DONOR

by Rachael Crais Wagner

Donor.

Please won't someone just save my mother.

I know it's a lot to ask, but I would do it for yours'.

Someone I don't know, someone other.

Will the one you give be what cures?

Cut it out, put it in.

Will that make us whole again?

My mental health during this time began to deteriorate rapidly. Who of all of us is their best sane self in high school? No one I know. But still, I took it to another, very scary level. I started saying, "I don't expect to live past 35" (PKD usually expresses itself in your thirties). I started making up ways to kill myself in "cool" ways when I turned that age. Going out surfing a tsunami will always remain my favorite. Then, in my musings, the age that I was assigning my death to grew sooner and sooner. Until I started thinking about the now.

This testimony shouldn't leave you thinking that your PKD will make your children suicidal. I have lived with varying degrees of depression my whole life. But as with any other high school kid, it all hit the fan during that time. Already trying to find a place in the world, dealing with figuring out my sexual preferences, and struggling in my friend groups was not made any easier by this new stressor.

I became a self-injurer. Those poems were a cry for help in a way I didn't know yet how to express. How do you tell the woman who is not afraid of anything, you are afraid? I couldn't figure out how to walk that line, so I spiraled down with my mental health. Watching my mother deteriorate, slowly lose her color, be a little more tired than usual, all seemed like witnessing a slow death. One I thought I would be next in line for. My birthright, as it were.

The day my mother was going in for surgery (I can't honestly remember if it was kidney removal or transplant day), I was called to the office in the middle of the day. I flew into a panic, worrying that something awful had happened, my teenage brain supplying the idea that my mom might be dead. The assistant principal got a shock when she told me I was being reprimanded for trouble in a class, and I burst into tears and explained that I thought I was going to be told that my mom's surgery had complications. I ended up getting out of trouble easier than I would have otherwise, so something helpful came out of it, but clearly neither I nor my family realized how anxious I was.

Now that I am older, the frightening experience of all this medical trouble is in the past, and my mother's been doing well ever since receiving a transplant from a lovely co-worker who is now a part of the family. It's been sixteen years, but I still recall the mental trauma as if it was yesterday. My story shouldn't make you think that this process is going to forever scar your children, but instead I hope it will help you realize that their mental health is an important thing to pay attention to during this process.

Suggestions for Parents

Because of my own experience and my unique perspective, I have some suggestions for parents with children facing a situation as I did. From the beginning of the diagnosis, be as honest as you can! Just try to be as upfront as you can about the trials and tribulations you are about to face, taking into account the child's age, of course. For your older children, particularly the teenagers, try very hard not to sugarcoat the information. Having a healthy optimism is important, but so is having your children not feel as if you're sweeping bad realities under the rug or hiding the seriousness from them.

By the way, if you have one meeting with your kids and it goes well, that doesn't mean you shouldn't check in with them again periodically to see if any new fears or concerns have reared up. Remember that no question is too silly. The better they understand the disease causing the need for a transplant, the less insecure they'll probably feel. If you think they can handle it, and you feel comfortable with it, bringing them into the room when the doctors describe treatment or transplant options could be helpful.

I also suggest watching out for any mood swings or unusual behavior. I know, I just summed up teenagers in their entirety, but erratic behavior could be directly related to the medical news. My depression absolutely took a turn for the worse once I heard the news. As someone who was very outgoing, I became more and more likely to shut myself in my room and eschew going out to dinner and doing family-related activities. I'm not sure if my teachers or school counselors were aware of my mom's condition before the incident with the assistant principal, but keeping your children's school support system aware is probably a great idea. They can be helpful watchers, keeping their eyes out for trouble. Additionally, giving the school a heads-up might prevent situations that could scare the kids, and help them have an easier time.

Suggestions for Teens

If you are a teenager facing a family member's kidney disease or transplant, I have some suggestions for you too. Ask questions when you need answers, but understand that you may have to do some of your own research. Your loved ones may not feel up to answering more invasive questions, but try to impress upon them that without knowledge you are left wondering and worrying. We live in an age where research is a lot easier to do than it used to be. If you use the Internet, try to stick to websites that are connected with well-known transplant centers—there is a lot of misinformation out there. If you're afraid, tell someone! Even a close friend can help assuage your fears a little. Do not try to face this by yourself as I did. You'll never get answers if you don't ask questions, and you won't get any comfort without conveying your fears.

When my mom first brought up writing this book, I was foolishly unsure about it. I know that she's written in scientific journals and has plenty of things published, but that's a very different type of literature. How could I have expected her to take to this like a duck to water? I should have known. Being an expert on almost everything, she took this on as she takes on everything: with strength, determination, and courage. I am glad she asked me to be a small part of the book and share my experiences here. I wanted to shed some light on the problems children might face with this sobering disease and the possibility of a transplant in the family.

I don't know if I have it. I haven't been tested yet. With all the uproar lately about insurance and pre-existing conditions, I'm nervous about getting tested and afraid to find out. But if I do have it, at least I know that I will have my mother to turn to when I have questions of my own.

Good luck to you in your journeys with this awful disease. Take mental health days when you need to, just don't forget that sometimes your kids might need some too.

Rachael Crais Wagner is a special-effects makeup artist in Los Angeles.

CHAPTER 15

When Even Family Donation Is Uncommon

Whether you're 15 or 35, seeing your strong, active parent suddenly in need can be devastating. Communication and particular cultural issues may add to the stress.

by Monica Sheppard

Recipient: Robin Williams
Date of donation: July 15, 2008 (second transplant, March 11, 2020)
Relationship: daughter
Location: Harrisburg, Pennsylvania

ORGAN AND TISSUE DONATION ARE uncommon in the African American community, largely due to misinformation and to the pervasive myth that treatment will be withheld if a designated donor is in the hospital seeking life-saving treatment. Years ago when my brother passed away, some family members believed he was not "saved" because of his organ-donor designation (even though he'd had a nonsurvivable brain injury). Given that history, I was certain there would be people among my family and close friends who would be worried about my decision to donate to my mother, but though there was concern, not one person disagreed. In fact, talking through their concerns made people want to learn more about living donation.

My kidney donation journey began in 2008 when my mom had just turned fifty-six. She'd suffered from hypertension and diabetes for years, and in 2007 was diagnosed with a somewhat rare kidney disease, FSGS (focal segmental glomerulosclerosis). The condition had led to end-stage renal disease. Once she had digested this information, my mom called to tell me, calmly and unemotionally. She said her treatment options were eventually going on dialysis or receiving a kidney transplant. Being highly emotional about matters that affected her was just not her way. She probably had concerns and fears that she never expressed to me.

My mom has always been a guarded and private person, so it was no surprise to learn she hadn't told anyone the news right away. I was stunned to learn of her diagnosis, though, because she was very active and didn't appear to have any major medical issues. (Later I realized that years of improperly managed hypertension and diabetes likely contributed to her kidney disease.) She wasn't prone to illness and, even when she did get sick, always pushed through and didn't allow much to slow her down. I immediately asked what I had to do to be tested. She informed me, and later my younger brother, that anyone could get tested if we were willing, to see if we were a match; in the meantime, she could get on the waiting list for a kidney from a deceased donor. Because I worked part-time as a social worker in the transplant community, I was all too aware of the amount of time people spend on kidney transplant waiting lists. In 2008 the typical wait averaged three to five years, often the latter. That would have almost definitely meant time on dialysis—and I did not want that for her.

I never wavered in my decision to donate to my mom. In fact, I urged her from that very first conversation to let the transplant center know I wanted to be tested as soon as possible. She has been the ultimate example of a giver, and I grew up seeing her give in so many ways, at times to her own detriment.

My mother was also a great supporter of all manner of donations. Years before her diagnosis she had donated bone marrow to a young teenaged boy she'd never met. She'd been tested and registered with the Bone Marrow Donor registry and was called to donate. It wasn't without discomfort, but she did so willingly and with a joyful spirit. When asked why she'd donated, she responded, "Why wouldn't I?! If given the opportunity to save someone's life without risk to their own, why wouldn't anyone?"

In 1995 she was again involved in making the decision to help people through life-saving donation. My brother Scottie tragically lost his battle with bipolar disorder (then called manic depression) and died through a self-inflicted gunshot. Scottie was a protective older brother and my very first best friend. We believed as a family that it would be a blessing to allow our tragedy to give others the chance at a better life by honoring his wish to be an organ donor. The Gift of Life donor program at Hershey Medical Center thankfully provided us with that opportunity. I continue to miss Scottie to this day but remain proud that he could help six others through organ donation.

Meeting one of my brother's kidney recipients that year was a moving and also a funny experience. A young white man, Wayne was shocked to learn that his donor was African American. He said that the doctor had told him he couldn't have had a better match in his own family, so he'd just assumed his donor was a young white man.

Although Scottie was registered as a donor, at the time my mom still had to give her consent, which she did without hesitation. The deceased organ donation process is longer than one might expect—at least a full day—because of the testing and matching. My mom was exhausted and grieving the loss of her oldest child at twenty-five, but she graciously allowed the center the time it needed.

After all those experiences, offering my mom the opportunity of a greater life was obviously a no-brainer for me. Giving her a part of me really was the least I could do. My decision was also selfishly motivated: I wasn't ready to face the thought of living without my mom at her best. Yes, I was in my thirties, and married, but who still doesn't want and need their mom? She cautioned me to take time to think about donation and discuss it with my husband, Reggie. Knowing the type of man Reggie is, I had no doubt he'd be nothing but supportive. I'd given him all of the information I could find on living donation, including risks, and he continued to support and encourage me. When I told him my mom had been concerned about his reaction, he said, "Why wouldn't you donate if you could help save her life? You definitely should do it!"

Several people wanted to know more about the living donation process, and were concerned about risks for me, which fostered some great dialogue. Some people told me they would never have considered donation before my experience because they didn't know a lot about it, but now they would. My dad was probably the most uneasy about the risks, and it took several conversations to allay his fears. One of his concerns was what it might mean if I wanted to have kids at some point (which I didn't, but there was no reason I couldn't). He and my mom had been divorced for years but maintained a closer-than-usual relationship for the sake of their children and grandchildren, so he absolutely had no misgivings about my decision to donate to her. As my parent, he just wanted to ensure that donating would not negatively affect me. Once his questions were adequately answered, he too provided unwavering support. In addition, my other brother decided that he wanted to also be considered for donation, and my father gave his blessing for him too.

My brother and I attended a comprehensive living donor transplant seminar at what was then Harrisburg Hospital in Pennsylvania. The transplant center required the orientation before any compatibility testing was approved. The several-hour seminar covered expectations and responsibilities for both potential donors and recipients, to ensure that everyone involved was knowledgeable before making such a big decision. About twelve to fifteen sets of patients and potential living donors attended, and they asked many thoughtful questions. A donor was on hand to answer questions about her experience, which was really helpful.

After the testing, my brother and I were given the news: he wasn't a match but I was. We also later discovered that he had risk factors that would not have allowed him to donate a kidney because of an increased likelihood of his having similar kidney problems later in life. I was asked to complete a multitude of physical and mental health screenings to make sure I not only was a physical match but also mentally capable of making such a difficult and life-changing decision.

I've always struggled with my weight, and I learned that I might have to meet strict BMI guidelines to be considered a viable candidate. I worried about this and thought that of all the criteria, this one might be an issue for me. But the transplant coordinator told me that overall physical health, risk factors, and activity level were taken into consideration and that I should be fine. Still, it definitely put pressure on me to watch my weight and exercise leading up to the surgery. I remember thinking I would be mortified if I was told I couldn't donate because of my weight, so that was an unanticipated stressor for me.

About two months after we began the testing, my mom started to experience symptoms of declining kidney function. She was not put on dialysis yet, but she and her doctors could clearly see the toll her decline was having and were eager to finish the testing so she could have the transplant. In spring 2008 we were finally given a transplant surgery date in May. A few days before our scheduled surgery, we were told that my mom's antibodies were unusually high and she would be the first in the transplant center to undergo plasmapheresis, a process that replaces the affected plasma to reduce high antibodies pre-transplant. The transplant would have to be delayed. Because the treatment was still so new, the transplant program had to fly in a plasmapheresis technician to administer it. We were naturally concerned and disappointed about the antibody issue and postponed surgery, but the delay was a blessing in disguise. My husband was in a pretty serious car accident four days before the first surgery date and wasn't in any position to help care for me after surgery as planned. My family and most of my closest friends lived eighty miles away in Harrisburg. And although Reggie's family lived within thirty minutes of us, they were very busy with their immediate families and their jobs.

After the first round of plasmapheresis, we were given a second surgery date in June. Once again my mom's antibodies were too high, so she underwent another round. The second treatment worked, and we were blessed with the opportunity to have our transplant on July 15, 2008. During the months leading up to the surgery, my mom's health continued to decline, and she was plagued with extreme fatigue to the point that she needed help even with minor tasks the week before the surgery. The night before was especially difficult, and she needed help to prepare for the next day.

On the day of the transplant, the hospital prepped my mom and me together, and my husband and several family members and friends were on hand to pray for us and wish us well. I cried for the first time in the process as they were wheeling me back to the OR—I wasn't afraid, but I was worried that this would not work as planned given the problems we had experienced leading up to surgery. A few hours later I was told my surgery had gone very well, that my kidney was a big "super kidney," and that my mom was currently in surgery receiving the gift. I was thankful, relieved … and hungry! My incision was about 2.5 inches on the right-hand side of my abdomen, and my pain was easily controlled with pain medication. I was able to walk the next day and to easily get in and out of bed on my own. The most difficulty I had was getting all of my systems to start working again.

My mom came through her surgery very well. Like most transplant patients, she immediately felt better after the transplant. It was obvious by her color, ability to produce urine, and energy surge that the surgery was a success. Our family was elated! We were in rooms across the hall from one another, and our family and friends wore a path across the hall checking on us.

I was discharged a day or two before my mom, and again I felt a strong sense of emotion as I prepared to go home to Maryland. As her only daughter, I instinctively wanted to stay to help her through her recovery period, but I knew that I needed time to recover properly myself and that she would be well taken care of by her sister, other family, and friends.

Days, weeks, and months passed and my mom continued to thrive. She was able to resume her fast-paced life and enjoy every minute of it. But like all things worth having, the transplant was not without some challenges. My mom had to take very high levels of immunosuppressants and other medications daily that all came with their own side effects. Since she was highly susceptible to infections, she was not approved to go to many public places for months after the transplant, including church. That was probably the most surprising and difficult challenge early on, because she was thankful and wanted to go to church to worship and praise God for the blessings. But the restrictions made complete sense and she abided by them. Eventually the safety precautions were lifted, and my mother was able to enjoy all of the things she'd enjoyed before the transplant. She and I benefited from the transplant in other ways too. We'd always been relatively close, but the transplant seemed to connect us in a special way, and we began to celebrate our T-day each July 15.

Things forever changed for us in late 2014. That September the transplant center gave my mom a clean bill of health; her creatinine level was really good, and by all accounts "the kidney" was doing well. However, the following month she began to get sick. On November 14 (my birthday) she was told that the kidney was no longer functional. She would need dialysis right away—and for the rest of her life. To say it was a blow to our entire family is an understatement. We were shocked, saddened, angry … we felt every emotion imaginable. But like all events to date in this journey, we accepted it and decided to push through the best way we could: with prayer, patience, love, and understanding.

The doctors don't know why my mom rejected that kidney. What I do know for sure is this: if I had been asked before the transplant if I would give her the kidney knowing that its shelf life would be six years, the answer without hesitation would be yes. Because I know for certain that the kidney helped her to lead a better quality of life for those six years that she might not have had otherwise. I had to remind myself and others of that as people expressed their disappointment and sadness for me. It was a shock, but we all knew of the risk. Now I will forever be a part of my mom, given that the kidney remains intact—just not functional.

In January 2020 my mom was approved to be on the waiting list for a kidney and gratefully received one from a deceased donor on March 11, 2020! That was in the beginning stages of the COVID-19 pandemic, so her hospital and home recovery looked a little different than usual. Since she didn't use any pain medication post transplant, my mom was advised to recover by herself if possible, to avoid the risk of any of us exposing her to the coronavirus. She had a visiting nurse come to the house for biweekly blood draws and had telehealth visits with her doctors instead of transplant clinic appointments. She continues to do well.

Whatever happens, donating a kidney to my mom was one of the greatest blessings in my life, and I would do it again in a heartbeat.

Monica Sheppard is a research analyst who lives with her husband in the Baltimore area.

CHAPTER 16

When the Donor Is the Partner

Even in families that are already knowledgeable about kidney donation, fear and other emotions can have a big impact on decision making when facing a health crisis. This couple, though both medical professionals, believe that they had long been in denial about the wife's kidney failure.

by Daniel Ranch

Recipient: Kanapa Kornsawad
Date of donation: April 28, 2009
Relationship: spouse
Location: San Francisco

KANA WOKE ME UP.

"I don't feel well."

"Should we go to the E.R.?"

We were both physicians, so we knew what that would result in: hospital admission, catheter placement, and hemodialysis. After several years of living with her chronic kidney disease, our transplant surgery date—and my donation—was now only three months away, yet it still seemed like an eternity. As we silently pondered the options once again, my mind took me back to how it all began.

Kana and I were in medical school in Bangkok when she began to complain of abdominal and back pain. She had brought up her symptoms to the professor, who proceeded to have another medical student demonstrate the abdominal physical examination on her in front of the class. She was eventually seen in the ER and had a urinalysis, which showed microscopic hematuria (blood in her urine). She was told she might have a kidney stone, and her symptoms eventually resolved. About a month later, Kana noticed small red skin spots on her forearms and ankles, so a skin biopsy was performed; it revealed inflammation of blood vessels in the skin. However, her testing came back negative, she did not develop further symptoms, and we were sucked back into the whirlwind of being medical students.

We were in the middle of our clinical rotations when Kana had her first kidney biopsy. She had not had any further follow-up on her hematuria, being bogged down with our training. One day she noted some leg swelling. A repeat urinalysis showed blood and protein in the urine. One of our favorite attending physicians, who happened to be a nephrologist, recommended that a kidney biopsy be done. There was no ultrasound guidance, just some local anesthetic and steady hands. We felt fortunate that this attending had agreed to do the procedure. Luckily afterward, Kana did not urinate blood or require a blood transfusion, complications we had seen a patient suffer after being biopsied by another physician.

The biopsy results showed IgA nephropathy, and we were torn between two different treatment recommendations. One physician felt that ACE inhibitor therapy and close monitoring would be appropriate. A different nephrologist strongly felt that Kana should drop out of medical school and start intensive steroid therapy. Even though both recommendations were valid at the time, the latter physician unfortunately was rude and demeaning. This fact, plus the specter of Kana having to give up her dream of becoming a doctor, turned us away from this course. Kana was started on an ACE inhibitor, and the issue once again fell by the wayside, as we continued our hundred-plus-hour weeks of medical rotations.

After graduating from medical school in Thailand, we decided to explore our training options in the United States. Kana and I had to live apart for a year when she spent time in a rural hospital as part of her loan repayment, while I stayed in Bangkok to study for the U.S. medical licensing exams. Kana recalls long days of seeing fifty or more patients in the morning clinic, then rounding on another twenty-five to fifty in the hospital wards. She exhibited intermittent leg swelling and had blood tests done once that revealed a serum creatinine of 1.8—almost twice the normal expected value. "That's normal, you're fine," she was told. We believed it, because that was normal for many patients in Thailand, which did not have the means to support chronic dialysis.

Kana and I then moved to the U.S., since I had matched into a pediatrics residency program in Las Vegas. A year later, my new friends and I were congratulating Kana for matching into an internal medicine residency program at the same institution. However, six months into her training Kana was found to have worsening kidney disease, and a repeat kidney biopsy showed progression of her disease. She was started on a course of oral steroids, and suffered through the typical side effects, including weight gain, facial acne, insomnia, fatigue, and mood swings. Like most people in denial, we eventually abandoned our own excellent nephrologist and went searching for other opinions. Kana and I were just hoping to hear someone say something different, that the IgA nephropathy wasn't getting worse, and that there was a treatment available or something we could try. In hindsight, we know very well how futile our actions were. But doctors are human too, and in times of crisis we will cling to any shred of hope, same as anyone else. Kana had withdrawn from her internal medicine training program, but we were surrounded by great people and eventual lifelong friends, who helped ease the pain. I ironically had matched into a prestigious pediatric nephrology fellowship program at UCSF in San Francisco, and soon we were on the move again.

Our luck and timing could not have been more perfect. This period was truly the first time that kidney transplantation had been a serious discussion. Kana and I had known for some time that we were a blood-type match and that a transplant was a distant possibility. However, we found that being under the care of a transplant center, there was an exceptionally different mindset and culture. From the beginning of our care there, the team's clear goal for us was a preemptive living-donor kidney transplant. Kana recalls crying with her parents over the phone, when telling them that I might be able to donate. It was a pleasant change from the usual "let's start dialysis, then see if you're a suitable transplant candidate, yada yada yada." This experience echoes the unfortunate concerns over inadequate education on the option of kidney transplantation compared to dialysis in new-onset ESRD patients.

And so that night that Kana woke me up, like many other nights, we decided once again to tough it out. Kana fought through her kidney failure symptoms, that general feeling of uneasiness, the hypersalivation and metallic taste in her mouth, and the migraines, for many months. She continued to battle symptoms that not all physicians are typically aware of, such as persistent fatigue, or the severe muscle cramping with toothbrushing or walking. Her driving force was that her transplant was around the corner, and that she could return to her medical training afterward.

The pre–kidney transplant evaluation team was wonderful. The coordinators were especially great, and really helped to put us at ease regarding the process. The difficult part for me was the actual testing, which in hindsight was even more nerve-wracking than the surgery itself. There was always the possibility that the team would find something which would preclude me from being Kana's donor, and this terrifying thought lingered throughout my evaluation. I recall having significantly high blood pressures at my initial visit, which turned out to be bad white-coat hypertension. My twenty-four-hour blood pressure monitoring test was completely normal. I also had a borderline-high serum creatinine, and I was unable to correctly complete a twenty-four-hour urine collection on two occasions. This was rather embarrassing for a nephrologist. But once again, I was exonerated with a normal blood GFR (kidney function) testing result. Finally, I had a CT scan done to assess my abdominal and vascular anatomy. I was relieved to hear that I had two normal-appearing kidneys; however, my left kidney had an extra renal artery, which meant that my right kidney would be the candidate organ. That said, I was good to go.

Thinking back, Kana and I had progressed through the Kübler-Ross five stages of grief (denial, anger, bargaining, depression, acceptance), although the process had taken several years. We had spent years turning a blind eye to the problem, despite having cutting-edge medical knowledge at our disposal. We blamed our doctors for bad news, and retained only the more hopeful parts. Kana and I prayed every night, hoping that this "madness" would miraculously just stop and disappear. Once we had exhausted all of our hopeless theories, that was when the feeling of defeat set in. I imagine it is this very same feeling that our patients suffer when they are given a grave diagnosis like kidney failure. Yet we were in the fortunate circumstances of being able to see the more encouraging option of transplantation, whereas most patients with kidney failure are still presented with dialysis as the next step. Having her transplant planned and ready to go was what helped us quickly accept our situation, years after it had begun. The last few months before the transplant, Kana and I were actually upbeat despite some of the rough nights she had to endure. I was settling into my training, and Kana was fortunate to have been hired as a part-time research coordinator with the department.

On the night before the transplant, I recall sleeping rather well despite the prospect of surgery the next day. By that time I had cared for many patients undergoing their own kidney transplants, although they were kids and their parents. That experience is probably what helped to put my mind at ease. Knowing what to expect definitely makes things less scary. Despite this, the morning of our surgery was a blur. We had checked into the hospital, with Kana's parents and my father and sister in tow. We settled into our respective rooms to change into our hospital gowns. Kana and I recall laughing when we saw how silly we looked in those gowns, and taking several comical pictures with our family and the delightful hospital staff. When we made it to the pre-operative area, I got to see Kana and say "I love you" one more time. The last thing I remember was the intravenous medication being pushed. Kana recalls becoming anxious once I was sedated, but she was comforted by her parents. It was not long before she was asleep as well.

In the recovery suite, Kana was awakened by the pain from her incision. She recalls asking for me, then fell back to sleep after being told I was fine. I remember waking up and having trouble catching my breath. The extra anxiety from not being able to see without my contact lenses probably did not help. My surgeon came by to check on me, and he told me I was fine. We now argue about who was the first to get up and visit the other, since it has been so many years. Kana recalls noticing that her legs weren't swollen anymore, and that the "fog" that had clouded her mind for so long had finally been lifted. The transplant team was happy with our recovery, and we were both out of the hospital after just three days, an amazing feat in hindsight.

The first few weeks after returning home were rather boring. Other than Kana's scheduled clinic visits, which were always quick and efficient, we didn't move much. We recall trying our hardest not to cough, sneeze, or laugh, since the extra pressure on our wounds caused pain. Kana's mother stayed with us for the first couple of weeks to help out. We invented several new techniques for rolling out of bed or climbing off the sofa. Fortunately, the pain improved soon after and we were back to walking or light gym training after the first five to six weeks. Kana had her energy back and felt great; I was back in the research lab continuing my fellowship research projects that had been on hold; being stuck at home watching daytime television had gotten rather dull. A few months afterward, we felt as if our lives had returned to normal.

Kana will never forget her nephrologists, transplant coordinators, and staff, and the wonderful care they provided. She is now an assistant professor in internal medicine at our medical school, and to this day she credits them for enabling her to achieve her dream of becoming a doctor. Every time her phone alarm goes off to prompt her to take her medications, twice a day at 8 a.m. and 8 p.m., we get a reminder about the remarkable events that happened. In retrospect, it was incredible how we were able to make it from advanced chronic kidney disease to living-donor transplant so smoothly, relatively speaking. As Kana and I both currently care for transplant patients in our respective careers, it makes us appreciate even more the great lengths that transplant teams have to go through for a successful living-donor transplant. We just wish that more patients with progressive kidney failure could follow our route and receive a preemptive kidney transplant, instead of having to start dialysis or endure the transplant waiting list.

We sometimes wonder what would have happened if we had made different choices during our adventure. What if Kana had chosen to drop out of medical school and start treatment? What if she had sought treatment back when her kidney function was declining in Thailand? What if I hadn't applied for nephrology training or hadn't been accepted into the program at UCSF? One could speculate that maybe Kana's IgA nephropathy progression would have stabilized or improved, or that she would have been started on dialysis sooner, or that maybe she wouldn't have needed a transplant at all. In spite of all this, Kana and I have no regrets. We are blessed to be in good health, and are privileged to have the opportunity to share our experience in the hope of helping others who have the unfortunate burden of kidney disease.

Daniel Ranch is a pediatric nephrologist who lives in San Antonio, Texas, with his wife, Kana.

CHAPTER 17

Close Siblings Become Even Closer

A brother and sister who have always been close feel a particularly strong bond when serious health concerns become paramount. This family's open communication helped them all weather the life-changing experience of donation and transplant.

BIG BROTHER MIKE RECALLS
by Michael W. Collins

Recipient: Wendy Withers
Date of donation: March 21, 1996
Relationship: siblings
Location: Dallas

OUR MOTHER OFTEN TELLS THE story that when my little sister Wendy was diagnosed with nephritis at age six, I told her not to worry, I would give her a kidney when the time came. I was sixteen.

We are a close-knit family, even (or especially) in troubled times. I have two older adopted siblings (Clark and Lynda), three blood siblings (Dan, Laury, and Wendy), and a half-brother (Russell) we have recently had the pleasure of welcoming to the fold.

Thanks to good medical care and prodigious amounts of steroids, Wendy spent most of her childhood and early adulthood in remission. She married and had two bright and beautiful daughters. A divorce followed, but by 1993 things were looking up.

Then Wendy's kidneys finally failed. I learned of it in a call from my father telling me that she was in the hospital. As I hung up the phone, I realized that the time had likely come.

I was a translator and small business owner in Chapel Hill, North Carolina, less than two years into my career and with a wife, two small children, and a new mortgage. My other siblings were at similar points in their lives. Nevertheless, after my parents brought Wendy and her children back to Texas (where most of our family live), and the diagnosis was confirmed and dialysis initiated, all three of Wendy's blood siblings stepped forward to volunteer a kidney. It seemed we would have her back on her feet in no time.

How wrong we were. Wendy was quickly added to the list of potential transplant recipients, but there were troubling signs that we should have paid more attention to. At her appointments, the doctors kept reminding her that it might be a long time before a cadaver kidney was available, to which she always responded, "I have several potential sibling donors." We kept expecting to be called for testing. Whenever we asked, we would get a vague response about not being at that point yet. Meanwhile, Wendy went through several serious health scares.

More time passed, and we began to realize that if the family did not advocate for Wendy with this unit that seemed so overwhelmed, no transplant would take place. After a series of contentious phone calls, including my father threatening legal action, suddenly things began to move. Arrangements were finally made to test us three siblings for tissue matches.

My brother and sister matched on three out of six factors (antigens). I matched on all six. Given how alike Wendy and I are, we were not surprised. The transplant was scheduled for March 1996, and we began to make arrangements to travel to Texas.

People asked a good many questions about our decision—"our" decision, because my wife, Mimi, and our children were of course a part of it all.

Is your wife OK with this?

Surgery always carries risk; wouldn't it be better for your sister to wait for a cadaver kidney?

What about your new business? Can you afford to be gone for six to eight weeks in all?

Was it a hard decision to make overall?

Strangely, I found these questions easy to answer, although I think my interlocutors were sometimes skeptical. My wife and I see the world with very similar eyes. To us, family is paramount, and the thought of holding anything back when we could possibly help is anathema. As for the risks, I had done enough reading and consultation to know they were not massive but were real. I was also not looking forward to the poking and prodding that were to come with testing. I have always stayed as far from the healthcare system as possible unless absolutely necessary.

This qualified as absolutely necessary. That my sister and I were a perfect tissue match meant that she would have an excellent chance for many years of healthy life. All other doubts and questions paled against the chance that her life could be saved. Businesses can be started over. Discomforts pass into memory. But to lose my sister without having done everything I could to help was unthinkable.

So, this was the easiest decision I have ever made. And I knew that were the situation reversed, Wendy or any of my other siblings would have done the same thing for me in a heartbeat.

We arranged a house sitter, and I squared things away with my partners, who showed amazing understanding, albeit with a healthy dose of trepidation. Mimi left her job in a university lab, freeing her to provide emotional support for our family, but adding to our financial uncertainty. We knew we would be away for at least four weeks and had no idea how easy or difficult my recovery would be.

In 1996 there was no laparoscopic surgery. The noninvasive surgery that's standard for donors now would not have worked in my case anyway because of the unusual configuration of my renal arteries. To remove my left kidney, they had to do the traditional twelve- to fourteen-inch incision running from just under the ribcage on my back all the way around to within six inches or so of my navel. The recovery was said to be often long and painful.

At the time, Wendy was living with my sister Laury and her family. After thirteen months on dialysis, Wendy was suffering from insomnia. Mimi and I had a pallet on the floor in Laury's living room, while Wendy was sleeping (or usually not sleeping) in an adjacent family room with a TV that stayed on all night. Dialogue from old movies drifted in as we tried to sleep. The blue light of the TV suffused the lower floor of the house. To me, that was when the full force of what Wendy was going through hit me.

By then, preparations were finally taking place with something akin to efficiency. Appointments were scheduled for Wendy and me to see the transplant surgeons, and for me to have a consultation, a physical, and other tests. These included a four-hour creatinine clearance test, an angiogram, and an arteriogram.

The frustration we experienced earlier picked up where our earlier struggles had left off. One day I had to wait almost eight hours for a physical examination. And there were interviews apparently intended to make sure I was psychologically healthy (including questions such as "Do you realize this is going to hurt?").

Early on, we had a consultation with the surgeon who would remove my kidney. He was a large man, and I couldn't help wondering how he was going to get those big hands inside me.

I recall undergoing a kind of angiogram with contrast medium injected in my arm. It was not sufficient, so I had to have an arteriogram as well. That was the single most unpleasant part of the whole process (including the actual surgery), mainly because I felt alert throughout the procedure, even though I believe I was supposed to be fully sedated.

The transplant was scheduled for March 1. We were both admitted to the hospital and taken through the informed consent procedure. Mimi was at my side every moment.

We were all mentally ready to go when the depressing news reached us the night before: the surgery had to be postponed. Wendy's liver inflammation values were elevated. We were discharged, and returned to Laury's home discouraged and unsure what to do.

They said it could be as much as several weeks before her liver values returned to normal. Should we go back to North Carolina and wait? Should we stay and hope for her rapid recovery? We decided to stay. I was afraid that if we left, we would lose the initiative and the transplant might never happen. We would stay for a couple more weeks and cut short the recovery time in Texas, meaning that if all went well, I would return home barely more than a week after the surgery.

Finally, Wendy's tests came back clear and the surgery was scheduled for March 21. We once again settled into our rooms on different floors, and the family shuttled back and forth between our rooms that afternoon and evening. Most of the attention was rightly on Wendy, as we were all nervous about the many things that could go wrong. By 1996 live-donor kidney transplantation was a fairly well refined procedure but still involved major surgery for both parties.

Early the next morning, I was taken to be prepped for the operation. Things were happening so fast, there was not really time to get nervous. They administered some anesthesia, and I began to get a little groggy.

When I woke up, the first thing I felt was freezing cold, despite the heated blankets. The recovery nurse provided the simple explanation: I had just spent a couple of hours split wide open in a cold room. No wonder the chill felt as if it had seeped into my very bones.

After some time in the recovery room, I was returned to my room and waited anxiously to hear how Wendy was doing. The surgeon came by and checked my dressing. All I could see of it was a long strip of opaque plastic material covering the roughly fourteen-inch incision running along my waist from my back to almost my navel.

I soon learned that everyone was a bit worried about Wendy's progress. The kidney was not working, and Wendy's spirits were reportedly low. While the situation was entirely out of my hands at this point, it was nevertheless discouraging to think it might all have been in vain.

As soon as it was OK'd, I was taken in a wheelchair to her room, where our whole family had gathered. Once there, we did what we always do when we are all together: we began joking, teasing, and laughing. For the two recently sutured surgery patients, however, every bout of laughter was immediately followed by a grimace and "ohhh!" which of course just made us laugh (and grimace) more.

A transfusion succeeded in jump-starting Wendy's new kidney. She immediately began to feel better and was discharged a few days later.

My stay passed without complications, but one moment stands out particularly clearly. A day or so after the surgery, the surgeon came by to inspect my incision. As he proceeded to strip away the plastic material covering the wound, I made an automatic defensive gesture to protect the wound, which the surgeon deftly—and coldly—blocked. I don't mean to imply he was insensitive—I liked him and felt he'd done an outstanding job. There was just something unsettling about being treated like a bystander in a situation I was intimately invested in.

Underneath the plastic strip was a terrifyingly long row of thick metal staples (the method of choice at the time) holding the two edges of the mother-of-all-incisions together, metal coming out on one side, looping over, and disappearing again into the other. However, everyone took a look and pronounced it good, and went about their business.

That night, I woke up tossing and turning, and couldn't seem to find a comfortable position. At some point the nurse came in and asked if everything was all right. I told her I was having a bit of trouble going back to sleep, and she looked at what I assume was a medications chart. "Oh!" she said, "you're in pain!" She returned shortly with a shot of Toradol, and I was able to sleep after that. Overall, however, I had remarkably little major discomfort, even though pain management was not as advanced then as it is today.

On day 5 post surgery, I was discharged with instructions to keep the wound dry. The staples were taken out a day or so before our scheduled return to North Carolina. The flight home was uneventful and I was back at my desk eleven days after the surgery. I should probably have waited a bit longer, but I had already been away for six weeks, and was eager to get back to business. I was not given any prescription pain medicine, nor did I feel I needed any, and there were no post-surgery tests or procedures except for a twenty-four-hour creatinine clearance test about six months after the surgery.

That test showed absolutely no abnormalities, and my health has remained excellent since then. I experienced some itching as the scar healed and a bit of numbness over the years, but nothing rising to the level of bother. Mimi and I have maintained an active lifestyle that includes biking sixty to a hundred miles a week, yoga, and travel. Not once have I felt that the kidney donation impaired my lifestyle in any way. Quite the contrary: I often forget for months at a time that it even took place.

As for Wendy, that is the best news of all. Thanks to the miracles of modern medicine (and a perfect tissue match!), the choice of how she wants to live her life has been placed firmly back in her own hands, and she has exploited it in spades. She has remarried, has several beautiful grandchildren, and is a consummate and highly respected professional, and one of the finest and most solid people I know. The kidney has continued to function flawlessly. It is truly the best outcome we could have hoped for.

It is strange to contemplate how we are able to live through such cataclysmic periods, fraught with pain, despair, fear of the unknown, just to have the pain fade away, leaving only the humor and warmth. I am so grateful for the support and understanding of my family and my extended family as we navigated those difficult times. But the decision to donate was never in doubt.

Mike Collins is a linguist and technical translator in Chapel Hill, North Carolina, where he lives with his wife, Mimi.

"KID SISTER" WENDY RECALLS
by Wendy Withers

Donor: Michael Collins
Date of transplant: March 21, 1996
Relationship: Siblings
Location: Dallas

IN DECEMBER OF 1993, I called a friend to pick up my two young daughters and take them to their family child care home. I had a flu I just couldn't shake and an ear infection, and I had spent most of the weekend incoherent and unable to get out of bed. So, I was headed to my doctor's office. Needless to say, I was shocked when after some testing, my doctor informed me that I was in end-stage renal disease (ESRD) and would soon be starting dialysis. I eventually would need a kidney transplant.

The day that I learned I had ESRD was one of the worst days of my life. I had been diagnosed with a form of IgA nephropathy, also known as Berger's disease, or nephritis, when I was six years old. Not knowing what it felt like to feel good, I took my state of health for granted. After the birth of my second daughter, however, my health began to deteriorate rapidly.

My husband and I separated when my youngest was three years old, and I was living in Omaha, far from my family and friends. My parents and older sister encouraged me to bring my daughters home to Texas and let my family care for me. And so I packed up our home and with my two daughters, who were six and three at the time, headed back to Corsicana to live with my parents. Unfortunately, the nearest dialysis clinic was approximately fifty miles away. Although initially I felt good as the toxins were cleared from my body, eventually the burden of every-other-day dialysis began to take its toll. I was exhausted, bruised, and sick most of the time.

Over the next fifteen months, to avoid the long trips to and from the dialysis center, I tried peritoneal dialysis at home, and various treatments to solve complications that arose from the dialysis. I suffered through an infection (peritonitis), low blood cell counts, nephropathy, and a host of other frightening issues.

Meanwhile we tried to start the process for me to get a kidney transplant. My pretreatment care and the arrangements for the transplant were handled by a national foundation, located near the transplant center where the transplant and donation were done. Even though I told them I had three potential kidney donors (my siblings), the hospital continually postponed the evaluations and so, my transplant. Nearly a year after my kidneys failed, my two brothers and sister finally were all tested and qualified as donors; one of my brothers, Mike, was a perfect genetic match, so he was the one who was going to donate to me.

Because my health was continually declining, after all the delays my father contacted the hospital and demanded that they schedule the surgery. During this time, I had moved to Denton, Texas, about fifty miles northwest of Dallas, to stay with my sister Laury and her children so that I could attend the University of North Texas and take advantage of educational benefits for individuals with disabilities.

When the date of the surgery was finally placed on the calendar, my brother Mike and his family flew in from North Carolina. He and his wife, Mimi, also had two little girls. This was naturally an extremely stressful time for everyone. I will be indebted to my sister-in-law forever for her patience and willingness to uproot her family for what turned into nearly two months as surgery was postponed because of my health problems.

There was a large group of us under one roof: my sister and her three children; my brother, his wife, and their girls; and my daughters and me. Not to mention dogs and cats and various other animals. Thank goodness for a big country farmhouse. Our family has always been quite close, and during that time we spent so many evenings and days together laughing and joking, making kidney jokes, and playing games. My parents would visit often, along with my other brother. It was a time when the world seemed to stop for a while as we waited in anticipation for the transplant surgery. We all grew closer as we prepared for the surgeries, one that we knew would cause my brother pain but ultimately would save my life.

When the day finally came, the Collins family took over the hospital by storm. We had wheelchair races in the halls, played cards, and laughed with family and friends as we waited. I remember waking up in the recovery room and hearing my sister comment that I was "pink"— the long days of dialysis had left my skin a sickly gray. I felt better that first day than I had in my entire life, after a transfusion got my new kidney working. I have never looked back since that day and have continued to feel better and stronger.

At that time, in 1996, the surgery for the donor was much more difficult than the surgery for the recipient. By then the donor organ was being surgically implanted in the groin area, spliced into the femoral artery. This reduced the amount of surgical trauma for the recipient. My brother stayed in the hospital longer than I did, and we all felt torn about leaving him in the hospital and going home.

In the end, the transplant process brought my family together in a way that is hard to describe. We were close to begin with and we all shared something special. Because of my brother's gift, I was able to raise my children and remarry; I have led a more-than-full life, graduating from college with my bachelor's degree, and completing a master's degree in public administration.

Best of all, largely because my brother's kidney was a so-called perfect match, after a few years my doctors decided to have me discontinue the antirejection medications that the vast majority of transplant recipients have to take for life. The doctors felt that the chances of rejection in my case were less than the chance of health-impairing side effects from the prolonged use of SandImmune. [*Important:* As tempting as the idea of discontinuing antirejection meds may sound to a kidney recipient, *stopping these medications can be extremely dangerous.* It's a very serious decision that only your nephrologist can make.]

I remain in great health twenty-five years after my transplant and enjoy camping, exercise, and baking. My brother Mike and I are still close and spend as much time together as possible, including a recent bicycle trip with the five Collins siblings. My husband and I have a son, three daughters, and seven beautiful grandchildren, whom I enjoy spending time with, and are currently raising four grand-nieces. I am eternally grateful for the generosity of my brother Mike and sister-in-law Mimi and the sacrifice they made to make this all possible.

For anyone who is considering giving the gift of life, I can assure you that it is a life-changing experience. It certainly changed mine.

Wendy Withers is city manager of the Town of Shady Shores, Texas, and lives with her husband in Krum, Texas.

Part Four: Community Connections

They're friends, neighbors, colleagues, faith-group members—
or just empathetic people who are moved by a story in a Facebook
post. Still others choose to donate to an unknown person they may
never meet. As more individuals share their stories of need,
more people learn that kidney donors and recipients don't have to be
related. As a result, though the idea may prompt concerns from their
loved ones, more nonrelated donors are coming forward.

CHAPTER 18

A Colleague in Need

by Linda Watson

Recipient: Elizabeth (Betsy) Crais
Date of donation: March 6, 2004
Relationship: colleague and friend
Location: Chapel Hill, North Carolina

BETSY AND I FIRST MET in 1988 when she was one of my professors in the master's program in speech and hearing sciences at the University of North Carolina at Chapel Hill, where I was a "nontraditional" (that is, older) student. Then in 1990, after completing my master's, I joined the faculty and we became colleagues. We worked closely together, and we became friends as well—which is true, I'm sure, for the vast majority of people who have gotten to know Betsy in any context, due to her outgoing personality and warm heart. Little did I know, though, that fourteen years later I would give her one of my kidneys.

I don't have any distinct memory of when I learned that Betsy had polycystic kidney disease (PKD). Among her colleagues, she was open about her diagnosis, but as a self-acknowledged wearer of rose-colored contact lenses, Betsy always maintained an optimistic outlook. I had not previously been close to anyone with kidney disease or otherwise had a reason to learn much about it. Thus, in part because of Betsy's optimistic perspective, I was very slow to understand the full significance of a PKD diagnosis, of Betsy's tests that indicated declining kidney function, or of her increasing number of kidney infections.

Then, in 2003, Betsy's doctors decided that a double nephrectomy was the best course of action to protect her health, and she had the surgery and went on dialysis. She tells her side of the story in this book. For me, this was the point at which I began to see what she was facing. For example, it was eye-opening to me to realize that she could no longer urinate, as happens to many people with kidney failure—it shouldn't have come as a shock to anyone who's had a basic biology class, but it really had never occurred to me before. I learned how carefully Betsy had to limit her water intake (along with other aspects of her diet) between trips to the clinic for dialysis, and then during dialysis, how often she had problems with swings in her blood pressure that raised other concerns.

The search for a kidney donor for Betsy was under way even before the nephrectomy. Again, reflecting my general ignorance of the topic, I did not realize that I might be an eligible donor. My impression was that if someone was unrelated to her, there would have to be a national search of a database of potential donors to find someone who would be a good match, with a small probability of finding one. Then I began to hear of the numerous nonfamily members who had volunteered to be evaluated as potential donors for Betsy. That so many people wanted to volunteer was a tribute to Betsy's generous spirit and the breadth and depth of her relationships. It also educated me that having a compatible blood type was the most important aspect of the match at the time, especially with the improvements in antirejection drugs.

One of these volunteers was another colleague of Betsy's and mine. She was tested and found not to be a viable donor, which was acutely disappointing to her. However, her stepping up to volunteer was what led me to consider it. I remember when I asked her what Betsy's blood type was and she replied, "A positive," as the point at which the seed was planted for me to become Betsy's donor. The more I thought about it, the more I felt compelled to volunteer to be evaluated. It just seemed that it was something I had to pursue.

Now I need to back up a little bit to talk about what was going on in my own life in 2003. Early that year, my eighty-one-year-old father had undergone a heart valve replacement and bypass surgery. Subsequently, complications from postsurgical infections led to additional major surgeries, and my smart, inquisitive father, who was known for his ability to consistently outwork people less than half his age, entered a period of rapid cognitive decline. We hoped that his cognitive issues might prove to be transient, but as the months went on, we had to face the reality that he was only getting worse. Although most of the burden of caring for him fell to my mother, my siblings and I tried to support them both as best we could. As one of their children who lived close by, I went to their home several times a week to, if nothing else, enable my mother to have a coherent conversation. Occasionally, I was rewarded with the feeling that I had made some connection with my father that gave him a few moments of pleasure. For the most part, though, he was angry and verbally (and sometimes physically) combative. Each visit added to my grief that I had already lost the father I had always known, to dementia if not yet to death.

Thus, I was sorely in need of some rose-colored lenses of my own around the time Betsy's health reached a critical point. So my decision to volunteer as her potential donor was driven both by my love for her as my friend and by my own need to do something life-affirming.

Now to pick up that story again. By the time I was ready to volunteer as a potential kidney donor for Betsy, at least two other people had started the evaluation process but had not been found eligible to donate. Knowing that Betsy was fighting to keep her optimistic perspective as she dealt with the challenges of dialysis, I did not want her to know that I was volunteering until I learned whether it would actually be possible for me to be her donor. So I contacted the coordinator of the donor program to see if I could be evaluated without Betsy's knowing. I knew that at least in our institution's program, only one potential donor could undergo testing at a time. When I contacted the coordinator, however, no one was undergoing active evaluation as a donor for Betsy, so I quietly began the testing process.

The testing started with a blood draw, filling up more test tubes than I had ever done before (even as a regular blood donor). My memory is not good for details about the evaluation process that occurred fifteen years ago. Obviously, everything proved to be fine in the end. But it was not a simple or short process. It seemed that each test left some question unanswered that required another test.

I remember that one early and basic test required twenty-four-hour urine collection. I had a basin for collecting the urine and a large jar to put it in. Then it had to go into the refrigerator. At that time, I had not told Mom that I was undergoing testing because I didn't want to cause her any additional worry before I knew whether I would actually be donating a kidney. On the day I had started the urine collection, my father ended up going into the hospital, so I went there to meet him and my mother. Several times during the day I had to make up an excuse to leave the hospital and drive the two miles home so I could urinate and store the urine in the refrigerator. Thank goodness my father was in a hospital close to our house! I think my mother was a bit mystified by my disappearances but was too concerned about my father to pry for an explanation. Along the way, I was tested to determine how balanced my kidneys were in their functioning, and had a kidney scan that required injecting a tracer into my veins. A psychological evaluation was required. And more blood tests. The testing procedures began to stretch out so long that the donor coordinator called me to say that Betsy was starting to wonder why none of the potential donors she knew about had started the evaluation process. She encouraged me to call Betsy and let her know that I was undergoing evaluation. Although still nervous about whether it was going to work out, I made that call, and Betsy was completely surprised. I told her that there was just one more test I had to have to confirm my eligibility, and that the transplant coordinator was fairly confident it would not prove to be a barrier. For my part, I was immensely relieved that the rest of the testing confirmed my eligibility to donate.

As the testing proceeded, I was impressed that after confirming the match as "good enough," most of the evaluation process was about determining whether I as the donor was healthy, was making the decision based on accurate information and without any pressure, and would be able to make the donation with a relatively low risk of experiencing any negative outcomes myself. Although I became impatient with the testing by the time I was approved, I ended up with lots of information that made me feel really good about my own health and firmly committed to donating a kidney to Betsy. And I had had plenty of time to think about it!

Perhaps I had acquired my own pair of rose-colored lenses along the way, because I truly never worried about experiencing problems related to the kidney donation. As many people would, I searched the Internet for information about kidney donation and also received a lot of information through the kidney donation program about the risks. Some of the information compared the risks of complications from donating a kidney to the risks of traveling by car. For many years, I have commuted more than fifty miles round trip between our home and my workplace, and the statistics made clear that I subjected myself to much greater risks many times over in my commuting than I would in donating a kidney. But the reality was that I had already made a decision in my heart about donating that had nothing to do with statistics about the risks.

My husband was less sanguine about my being a donor, however. It surprised me, because he is an engineer, and I thought he would be reassured by the risk statistics. Instead, all my father's medical complications had led my husband to assume that the worst possible outcome of any surgery would be almost inevitable. But he said that it was ultimately my decision, and I told him that I wanted to make the donation, not just for Betsy's sake but also for my own. Interestingly, when we went together to meet with the surgeon prior to the donation, the surgeon pulled up 3-D images from my kidney scan, and somehow seeing all the details in the images and hearing the surgeon's description of the procedure reduced my husband's anxiety in a way that no other information had been able to do. My mother had some concerns when I told her that I was going to make the donation, but I think she also welcomed the positive aspects of my decision in the context of the challenges and sadness our family was otherwise experiencing.

Betsy and I scheduled our surgeries for our spring break in 2004. A friend at my church who makes jewelry made bracelets for Betsy and me using beads from various stones associated with good health, and Betsy and I arrived at the hospital wearing our bracelets. My sister came from her home in Memphis to provide some extra help for my parents during the week of the surgery, and on the day of the surgery, Mom arranged for a caregiver to stay with my dad so that both she and my sister could be at the hospital with my husband. One funny thing I remember is that one of the doctors came in as I was being prepped for surgery and wanted to know where the rest of my chart was. Apparently, he was not accustomed to seeing surgery patients who did not have a fat medical folder to accompany them, but the only times I had ever been hospitalized were for giving birth to our two children. And they were adults by then.

Sometime after I had been moved from the surgery recovery area into a hospital room, a nurse asked me if I wanted to go down the hall to see Betsy. Of course I did! When I went in the room, there was a bag hanging from her bed filled with urine from her catheter. The doctor told me that my kidney had "pinked right up" when they transplanted it in her and started producing urine almost immediately. I would never have predicted that I could get emotional about seeing a bag full of urine, but I did. The closest feeling I can compare it to is the experience of the miraculous that I had when each of our children was born. For many months after the surgery, I felt grateful every time I urinated that my body allowed me to do that and also that Betsy's body would allow her again to do the same thing.

Betsy and her husband gave me a living gift of a redbud tree to com- memorate our emotional and physical connection, and it continues to bring a smile to my face each time I see it in our front yard. My left kidney is still work- ing in Betsy's body. I realize that she likely will need another transplant at some point, and I think I will feel a bit sad about the loss of my left kidney if and when that happens. But I also know that fifteen-plus years is a good amount of time for a donated kidney to function. And Betsy still has her rose-colored lenses on. One thing I do not worry about is whether there will be another volunteer to donate a kidney to her. As happened last time, I think people will be getting in line to express what she means to them in this way. Truly, we are the lucky ones to have her in our lives, helping all of us to more often see the world through rose-colored lenses.

Linda Watson is newly semiretired from her career as a professor of speech-language pathology and autism researcher; she lives with her husband in Raleigh, North Carolina.

CHAPTER 19

Potential Donors Found *Him*

by Joe Reichle

Donor: Robert Drager
Date of transplant: August 3, 2003
Relationship: friend
Location: Minneapolis

IN 1980, AT AGE TWENTY-NINE, I learned the news I had expected since I was sixteen: I had polycystic kidney disease (PKD). My father had died from it at fifty-four. His brother died from it soon after at about sixty. A third brother died from it several years later. Kidney transplants were not reimbursable through our insurance at the time. My family was relatively poor and did not have the resources (or perhaps the knowledge) to pursue a transplant. As a young teenager I just assumed, based on my family's experience, that I might die of the same disease sometime between fifty and sixty years of age. The story that follows suggests that although it hasn't always been smooth sailing, as I approach seventy in relatively good health, I've obviously benefited from opportunities I never expected.

I was diagnosed at the University of Vermont Medical Center where I was a brand-new faculty member. When I saw my general practitioner for an intestinal flu, he felt a mass near my kidney region. I remember overhearing the physicians discuss my test results before one of them came into the room. One said, "poor guy" (not exactly a confidence builder). My doctor referred me to a genetics specialist for counseling, which reinforced my worst fears. I assumed the geneticist was going to counsel me to strongly consider not having children because they might have the same disease. Sure enough, my pregnant wife and I were advised to consider the implications of having children—not the greatest timing. PKD results in a 50% chance that children will have the abnormality. We did not heed the advice, and my wife, Patti, and I have two children.

We moved to the University of Minnesota in 1981. I knew Minnesota had several well-regarded transplant centers, and I made an appointment at the university's renal clinic. Up to then, my experience with physicians had been very scary (completely unrelated to their competence). It just seemed that almost every time one of my relatives visited a physician, the result was very bad news.

My appointment with a nephrologist at the renal clinic was different from my previous experiences. The first question I asked was, "How long do you think I have to live?" His response was "I have no idea, but your tests are all very normal with the exception of those related to your kidney disease. If that remains the same, I'd say whatever the mean life expectancy is these days." I asked how he could say that, given the history that I had outlined. "We are no longer in the 1950s, Joe," he said. "We can do things to put you in a position to have a good and productive life."

I began to look forward to visits to my new friend. Given that I've always been a worrier, my perspective on life pretty much began a 180-degree turn. I concluded that the genetics counselor in Vermont had given me potentially bad advice. Over the next thirty years I led a normal life, had a successful career as a professor, and with my wife raised two wonderful children.

As we approached the mid- to late 1990s my fears began to reappear very gradually. My creatinine, which is a gross measure of kidney function derived from a blood sample, had been normal or close to normal (around 1.0–1.1) for quite some time but began to dramatically deteriorate. I began scanning websites about transplantation. I learned that when patients' creatinine reaches approximately 5.5, physicians usually begin to prepare them for dialysis. By 2003 mine had reached 5.8. However, each patient is different. My nephrologist had done a good job in "warning me up." He began providing details about the transplant process and had videos to illustrate what is done during surgery and what to expect after the transplant. Over more than a year, my checkups gradually went from yearly to every three months. By 2003 I was having labs done monthly and checking in with my transplant coordinator; I realized that I was bound for either dialysis or a transplant soon.

About then I began to have a few symptoms confirming that I was having some renal difficulty: a little nausea and an occasional slight metallic taste in my mouth. Once during my monthly checkup my nephrologist asked how many friends and relatives I had. He said that if I was willing, my wife or a friend might want to casually make them aware that my kidneys were failing and I'd need a transplant. My current and former doctoral students with whom I corresponded regularly knew my health status. Some of them began an email chain without my knowledge, explaining to others that my kidneys were failing and that I needed a transplant.

I am a person who doesn't like to ask for things. I had always assumed that if I got a new kidney it would be from a deceased donor. The wait for a deceased-donor organ was almost five years in my state. I was aware that a deceased-donor organ functioned substantially less long than a live donated organ. I also knew that being on dialysis prior to a transplant tended to reduce the longevity of the transplant. Each of these facts greatly heightened my anxiety about waiting for a deceased-donor kidney. Although I didn't like the feeling of being indebted, I knew that my quickest path to potentially longer survival required finding a live donor. Consequently, I allowed it to be made common knowledge that my kidneys were failing and I would have to go on dialysis soon. To my great surprise, as people began to learn of the urgency of my situation, the prospective donors seemed to find *me*. Three faculty colleagues contacted me to say that they had gone through donor testing. One told me that she was pretty sure she had been approved. However, further testing revealed that she had a slight kidney abnormality, and that it might not be in her own best interest to donate. The transplant committee did not approve her as a donor.

The colleague came to my office to give me the news, with a tear slowly making its way down a cheek. We had been good friends for years, and she had seen my health problems firsthand. I think she had been so sure she would be able to donate that the bad news was almost as crushing to her as it was to me. She repeatedly apologized. I've always thought of myself as a good person, but this single experience taught me that she was a far better person than I was. Not only was she willing to donate part of her body, but it made her extremely sad that she couldn't do it. My friend no longer lives in Minnesota, but fifteen years later we still communicate regularly. If anything, the experience made us better friends

The search for a kidney continued. I had a wonderful former doctoral student who offered to be my donor but later found out that she was pregnant. Fortunately, her husband volunteered to be my donor. I should mention that every transplant center has protocols to ensure that no coercion is taking place in an offer to donate. Because of our former student-faculty relationship, for either of them to donate to me might have represented a conflict of interest. However, her husband was cleared as my donor. At about the same time, I was supposed to see a surgeon who would be creating a dialysis port in my arm. Now that I had an approved donor, however, I was able to avoid that surgery and was transplanted without ever experiencing dialysis (known as a *preemptive transplant*).

Both my transplant surgery and my donor's surgery went well, with no complications for my donor but a few for me that I'll describe later. My kidney was working immediately and within hours my creatinine went from 5.8 before surgery to 0.9 (after a few days it settled into around 1.2). Within a day I was walking, and the nurses were telling me how many laps around the nursing station they wanted me to do. I was in the hospital for about five days. My pain was well controlled, but my first few days of immunosuppressants were literally gut wrenching. I felt nauseous or vomited fairly often after medication. I suspect that the pain medication was partly to blame. Soon my stomach settled down and I was feeling first-rate. I thought, "This is a breeze." After about three months I returned to limited teaching and by spring semester had pretty much assumed my prior responsibilities.

My nephrologist explained that although my case had gone smoothly, many transplant recipients have a few glitches along the way and I should be prepared for some ups and downs during my first year. Over a period of about six weeks into my transplant, I noticed a consistent increase in my creatinine level. My nephrologist said that a change of less than 0.3 or so wasn't really considered clinically significant. However, during a several-week period it went from 1.2 to 1.8, and my wife can attest that all I talked or read about was kidneys. I was looking for the standard range of measurement error in creatinine testing and how various factors influenced creatinine levels. I was drinking up to 85 ounces of water a day. I also engaged in superstitious behavior. If I had a good lab the day before, I called for lab results at the same time the next day. Of course, none of this helped. My lab data clearly displayed a downhill trend. I knew that there was some physician concern because my lab schedule changed from twice a week to daily.

My kind and knowledgeable transplant coordinator was wonderfully accessible. She checked in regularly and was available to discuss any problems. I consulted her so often, I feel extremely fortunate that she did not block my phone number. I was concerned that my labs were not maintaining their original post-transplant levels. She agreed that the trend could not be explained away. One day she called and told me to go to intervention radiology so they could see if fluid was building up around the kidney (hydronephrosis); she said that it might be necessary to do a kidney biopsy. I didn't need to ask why. A biopsy meant that they were suspecting rejection.

An ultrasound confirmed that I had hydronephrosis. It appeared that not all the fluid I was drinking was getting to my bladder in a timely fashion. Further tests confirmed that I had a narrowing of my new ureter, which had been crafted when I had my transplant. This, of course, was upsetting, and I immediately started panicking, again reading articles online and becoming a pest to my nephrologist and transplant coordinator. Fortunately, they recognized my concern and assured me that sometimes this happens and a procedure could be implemented that would preserve the new kidney. Without a well-functioning ureter, urine backs up in the kidney and if left untreated can cause significant damage and threaten the viability of the transplanted kidney.

I was not that familiar with intervention radiology. During my first visit the doctors inserted a stent in my ureter to hold it open. They also diverted urine from the kidney to a small bag worn on my leg. This was all done as an outpatient with no pain. I did this for a few months. Once the stent was inserted in my ureter, kidney function soon returned to normal. Since stent removal my kidney has functioned well. Although the stent solved my problem, it created some minor discomfort. Additionally, I had to wear that exterior urine bag.

One day a resident who replaced my catheter to the bag collecting urine affixed it incorrectly. This resulted in a very slow leak, which, unfortunately, my students in class noticed before I did—needless to say, this also resulted in a shortened class. I simply went back to radiology, where the leak was quickly solved.

After a transplant it is important to be regular in your medical visits. With a compromised immune system, it is much easier for infections to get started and spread. Always in the back of my mind is the knowledge that my chance of having a range of malignancies is increased because of my suppressed immune system. Also, PKD has a few associated conditions that can be life threatening (e.g., aneurysms). Given the range of potential medical issues that can occur, it's particularly important to find physicians who regularly read the literature in their field, are good listeners, and are not intimidated by lots of questions.

Except for occasional skin lesions, my health has been fine. My dermatologist suspects that these conditions are related to my transplant medications. I have had several instances of inflammation of the prostate gland and one or two urinary tract infections each year that require antibiotics. Within a day or two if not treated, my UTIs can result in a high fever and being in bed for several days. I was hospitalized with shingles several years ago and was on steroid and antiviral medications for a while after my hospitalization. Despite these anomalies, the vast majority of the days since my transplant have been spent in good health. My transplant has created no real restrictions.

I take a mix of two different immunosuppressants twice a day and several other medications to address high blood pressure due in part to my PKD.

I view my medications as a minor inconvenience compared with the problems I would be having without a transplant.

If I could have done anything differently, it would have been to discuss removing my native kidneys at the time of my transplant. My old kidneys no longer function and are essentially collections of large cysts that occasionally burst. This can be painful. They could also potentially become infected. The biggest problem is that together with my cystic liver (polycystic kidney and polycystic liver disease often go hand in hand), my internal organs take up a lot of space that gives me a larger-than-I'd-like belly. This, in turn, has resulted in an umbilical hernia, which at some point may require surgery.

Despite the minor setbacks and inconveniences mentioned, if your kidneys are failing, a transplant is not something to shy away from. It can dramatically improve your quality of life. As with any major surgery there are risks. However, the success rate is incredibly high. I think my experiences related here are probably not that different from those of a number of transplant recipients. For those of you who are candidates for a transplant, the odds are very good, and better than they've ever been, that it will work out very well for you, too.

Where We Are Today

My donor. Every day I am grateful to my donor, Robert Drager, his wife, Kathy, and their two fantastic kids. My wife and I have joined them for baseball games, river cruises, and pizza places with arcades. We have followed each other's family events—the happy ones and the sad ones.

My family. Both of our adult children are well and have declined to be genetically tested. As they approach the time in their lives when symptoms often begin to show for this disease, I have a renewed sense of anxiety until I remember that I've had sixty-nine great years with the disease, and with advances occurring, it's quite likely that their lifespans will be much longer than mine.

Me. I know that many people with polycystic kidney and liver disease are otherwise reasonably healthy and have full, productive lives. Having a transplant has reminded me to address the things that are most important and to worry less about small, day-to-day problems. At this writing, it has been seventeen years since my transplant. Statistically, I probably have fewer years left with it than the number of years it has been keeping me alive. This probability has increased recently with a diagnosis of polycythemia vera, a rare blood cancer that has no cure. Fortunately, for most individuals, it progresses slowly. Thus, I continue to forge ahead with what might best be described as "living on borrowed time."

Joe Reichle is professor emeritus of speech-language-hearing sciences at the University of Minnesota; he lives with his wife, Patti, in their home on Lake Michigan.

CHAPTER 20

He Donated to Someone
He Might Never Meet

by Brad Dean

Recipient: Sue Gommer

Date of donation: December 5, 2011

Relationship: nondirected donation

Location: Durham, North Carolina

"PERFECT MATCH." THOSE TWO WORDS uttered by an organ transplant special-ist elicited an indescribable combination of joy, excitement, anticipation, and anxiety. I was about to embark on a life-changing endeavor for me and three people I had never met.

My interest in organ donation had begun long before that day in 2011. I was continually amazed at the advances in modern medicine, saving lives with transplants of hearts, lungs, kidneys, and other vital organs. What once seemed like fantasy or science fiction had become semiroutine medical pro-cedure. Knowing generally the impact that organ donation could have on the lives of others, including my family, I always proudly signed up as an organ donor with each renewal of my driver's license.

But then the concept became very real and personal for me when two organ recipients touched my life in a very significant way. One was a co-worker whom I had known for many years, the other a professional acquaintance who had become a mentor to me. I came to realize that I had already benefited by organ donation through their impact on my life. In some ways, the man I am today was shaped by those individuals.

It was 2010, and I watched with great sadness as my dear friend and mentor slowly died from liver disease. He had received a liver transplant many years before and often encouraged me to support efforts to promote and fund organ donation. He would smile and gently remind me, "You never know whose life you might be saving." My friend needed a second liver transplant, but because of the long list of hopeful recipients and his deteriorating health, a transplant was unlikely. Because of our blood types, I knew there was no way I could be a donor for him. This was the first time I knew someone who died waiting for a transplant.

Around that same time, I was visiting a medical center for my annual physical. I had enjoyed good health up to that point and expected a positive report. The full-day exam included an endless battery of tests, and it would be an hour or two before my doctor could finish my exam, so I camped out in the nearby waiting area, under a sign reading "Dialysis Waiting Area."

What I observed astounded me. The room was filled with a cross-section of America: young and old, male and female, white and black. I had wrongly assumed dialysis mostly affected older adults in poor health, but seeing the faces in that room impressed upon me the broad impact of kidney disease. Every conversation I overheard centered around "waiting." Waiting for the doctor. Waiting for the nurse. Waiting for a transplant. But one patient spoke words that haunt me to this day.

He was a middle-aged man, not much older than I was. He wore a business suit and was reading the *Wall Street Journal* while he waited. He asked how long I had been receiving dialysis. I explained that I wasn't on dialysis; my health was fine, and I was simply waiting for the results of my annual physical. He paused, noted how fortunate I was, and solemnly recalled the days when his health was good. "But now," he said, "I'm just like the rest of these people—not living, just avoiding dying." *Just avoiding dying.* I could feel the frustration in his voice.

Soon, my doctor invited me into his office to discuss the results. I had confidently expected the positive report I received but now felt very grateful, even a little guilty. I asked, "How are my kidneys?" The question surprised him at first. He fumbled with the lab results for a few seconds, nodded his head, and said with a smile, "Your kidneys are perfectly healthy. You're lucky. I know people that would give anything to have just one healthy kidney, and you have two."

During my drive home, and for the next few days, I couldn't shake that experience. I had acquired an intense curiosity about kidney donation. I was amazed to find that many people live a perfectly healthy life with just one kidney. Transplants had become more common and less risky. Yet the need for kidney donations far exceeded the supply of healthy organs. People were dying while waiting for a donor. All the while, I could not forget those words: "not living, just avoiding dying."

The thought of donating one of my kidneys seemed outrageous, yet I couldn't get the idea out of my mind. I had two young children at home. What if something went wrong during the surgery? What if I acquired kidney disease afterward? Worse yet, what if one of my children ever needed a kidney and I was unable to donate? For the next few weeks, it seemed as if I couldn't read a newspaper or watch television without seeing something related to organ donation. All the while, I kept ignoring the internal pull to become a donor.

My Christian faith is the center point in my life. I knew all too well the Bible Scripture that teaches us "*Greater love hath no man than this, that a man lay down his life for his friends*" (John 15:13 KJV). I began to pray for direction. Well, actually, I prayed for God to take this desire away from me, but He didn't. The more I prayed, the more I felt compelled to donate.

I shared all of this with my wife, my father, and my pastor, half expecting one of them to talk me out of what still seemed like a crazy idea. They each offered their prayerful support and encouragement, reassuring me that if this was a desire God had laid on my heart, I was foolish to fight it. Over the next few weeks, I became increasingly at peace with the idea. I was now ready to commit to what was certain to be a monumental experience.

The professionals at the North Carolina medical center I chose are world-class. They take their jobs very seriously and excel in every aspect. I was familiar with the center's excellent reputation in healthcare and knew several people who credited it for saving their lives. From my research, it was clear that it was a leader in organ transplant, so I felt very comfortable volunteering for its transplant program.

To my surprise, evaluation of my mental and emotional state was every bit as important as my physical health to the medical team. They were exceedingly thorough and very frank in their assessments and reviews. At times, I felt they were discouraging me from being a donor. I realize now they were simply doing all they could to ensure that I was prepared physically, emotionally, and mentally for the task ahead.

I was now fully committed to becoming an altruistic donor—that is, a nondirected donor. This meant I might never meet my recipient. Some people find that odd, and admittedly it is a peculiar arrangement. But I found it to be advantageous. Had I learned that the recipient was a friend or family member, my Type A personality would have kicked in and I would have worried endlessly. What if we were not a perfect match? What if the transplant failed? Not knowing the recipient enabled me to focus on only those details I could control, putting the results in God's hands (who, in turn, worked through the very talented hands of some remarkable doctors and nurses at the transplant center).

Within a few weeks, I received a call explaining that I could choose to join the center's first paired transplant. A woman with kidney disease was desperately in need of a healthy kidney, and her daughter had volunteered to be a donor but was not a match. I was a match for the mother, so the daughter pledged her kidney to a man on the waiting list. I had spent months wondering if I should give a kidney to save one life, and now God was using me to help save two lives.

I had many doubts, right up to the day of the surgery, and so did others around me. When I shared my plans with family, friends, and co-workers, the responses were varied and unpredictable. Most were surprised, because I had not shared my desire to become a living donor with many people. Some were instantly supportive, while others were cautious and reserved. A few tried to talk me out of it, but by that point, my mind was made up. As a living donor, it's helpful to anticipate that those around you may react in different ways, and not to be alarmed by this.

Just three days before the surgery, I received a call from Neil Offen, then a reporter with the *Herald-Sun* in Durham, North Carolina (and the husband of this book's co-author Carol), who had been given my information by the transplant program. Medical professionals are required to protect a patient's privacy, and I had initially rejected any notion of publicizing my surgery. However, a friend observed that by sharing what I was about to do, I might prompt others to consider becoming an organ donor, which could save more lives. After much thought, I authorized the team to share my information.

Answering reporters' questions is part of my daily work as a chamber of commerce president, but this was different altogether. The reporter had spoken with the recipient, Sue. As he asked me various questions, I had to fight the urge to start interviewing him. What was she like? How old is she? Where does she live? Is she nervous? Relieved? How long had she waited for a donation? Up to this point, I knew virtually nothing about the lady with whom I would soon become inextricably linked.

Those last few days before the surgery are a blur to me. My work required steady travel and that was actually helpful. In the back of my mind, I grew increasingly concerned about something going wrong, and the conscientious transplant staff had been very candid about the risks of surgery. I made it a point to call many friends and colleagues, partly to invite their prayers and encouragement, but also to seize the opportunity to let them know how much they meant to me.

I don't think the magnitude of my decision to become a living donor fully hit me until that final goodbye before the surgery. My wife and I were departing for the hospital, and our children would stay behind. The notion that this could be the last time I held my kids overwhelmed me. We had explained the basics of organ donation, hoping they would see this as a selfless act of love. But my teenage son understood better than his younger sister the risk. Sharing age-appropriate information with your children is a key consideration for donors, and one that cannot be taken lightly. We were all hopeful, but nervous.

My wife had been resolute and strong in her support from the start. But now, we both sensed the significance of this decision not only for me, but our entire family. Doubt crept in and for the next few hours, my mind raced between proceeding with the kidney donation and calling the hospital to cancel the surgery. I couldn't erase the mental picture of my children looking at me with both pride and fear. But I also thought about the two recipients and their families, all of whom were now counting on me.

When my wife and I walked into the hospital, we were greeted just as any other patient is. I received a lengthy list of do's and don'ts, along with regulation hospital attire. I sat in the waiting room with several other patients who were also awaiting surgery. I wondered if those sitting near me included my kidney recipient, or perhaps the other donor-recipient pair (they did not). A continuous line of medical personnel attended to every detail and repeatedly asked me if I was certain I wanted to go through with the surgery. I think I must have been offered the opportunity to opt out at least a couple of dozen times that morning, right up to the point at which the anesthesiologist put me to sleep.

The surgery was uneventful, or so the doctors say. I say losing a kidney is anything but uneventful! I experienced much discomfort and had difficulty sleeping for the first few days. From the moment I awoke, I had a gnawing desire to know if the recipient was okay. Because of HIPAA and hospital protocol, the doctors and nurses refused to give me any details. I worried that the surgery had failed and became convinced the staff was avoiding telling me the bad news.

Eventually, I learned that both transplants were successful. All four of us—donors and recipients—were healing well. I felt relieved, and became intently focused on my recovery. I had my wife leave out my jogging shorts and running shoes in plain view, so I could keep my mind focused on where I was aiming—that is, full recovery. I didn't have much of an appetite, but with one kidney, I quickly become aware of the need to stay hydrated and eat healthy.

I didn't expect to meet Sue. I'd understood from the outset that I might never get to meet her or the others involved in the paired transplant. I left the hospital on the third day after the surgery, and that's when I was introduced to

Sue, her daughter Jennifer (the other donor), and Jeffrey (the other recipient). What a joy to see Sue's big grin and shining eyes! Words escaped us both. But the bond that was created—medically—had become much more when I was able to see her smile.

Within a few days after my release, I was walking two miles per day and soon thereafter I returned to work. Things were back to normal, although it was a new normal for me. No longer could I take for granted having healthy kidney function. I now pay specific attention to nutritional requirements and the importance of drinking lots of water. I am ever mindful of avoiding injuries to my remaining kidney.

Occasionally, I'm asked about my decision to donate a kidney. Some are considering becoming a donor and want my insights. Some have recently lost a kidney and want to know what life with one kidney is like. Some just simply want to know if I would do it all over again.

Undoubtedly, I would do it again, without hesitation or reservation. I would do it in honor of those organ recipients who have impacted my life. I would do it to faithfully follow the desire God put in my heart. I would do it to set an example for my children, that they might be inspired to live a life of generous giving. Most of all, I would do it simply to know that Sue, Jeffrey, and others like them can live an abundant life. That's far better than the alternative of "not living, just avoiding dying." If my sacrifice of one healthy organ can change the lives of those around me, it's worth it no matter the cost.

Brad Dean is a tourism executive who lives in San Juan, Puerto Rico, with his wife, Myriam.

Part Five:
Supporting Roles

*A dedicated group of people—transplant coordinators,
caregivers, donation advocates—closely help support living donors
and recipients through this remarkable process.*

CHAPTER 21

Helping Overcome Transplant Obstacles

by Tammy Wright

Tammy Wright is a transplant nurse coordinator at Sharp Memorial Hospital in San Diego; she has worked in transplant care for more than twenty-five years.

UNDER THE BEST OF CIRCUMSTANCES, the transplant and donation process can be stressful, with many ups and downs. It's particularly so when recipients who originally were compatible with their donor find on the repeat testing that they are no longer compatible, when either person becomes ill, or when a donor's family obligations make travel to the recipient's far-off transplant center unfeasible. Fortunately, in many cases these obstacles are surmountable—often through kidney paired exchange, or KPE—and these people are able to proceed with their living donation and transplant after all.

During a transplant evaluation, all potential recipients are encouraged to find a living donor—both to shorten the time they need to be on dialysis and to improve their prospects for better health. Even once a living donor has been identified, potential recipients may experience many frustrating stops and starts. Here are just a few examples of the many success stories that have touched and inspired me. (Some names and identifying characteristics have been changed to protect privacy.)

Lisa and Susan

Scheduling a kidney donation and transplant is a very delicate balance of needs and timing. Susan wanted to donate to her friend Lisa, who was born with diabetes that was causing her kidneys to fail. Because she still had some kidney function, Lisa was not on dialysis, and the transplant team wanted to wait to transplant her until her kidney function was lower but *before* she needed to start dialysis. She was put on the transplant waiting list. Susan completed the living-donor testing and was approved.

Six months later, when Lisa was ready for the transplant, a repeat cross-match showed that Susan and Lisa were no longer compatible. This was devastating news to both of them, especially because Lisa was starting to have more symptoms of kidney failure and was close to needing dialysis. In the past, we would have tried to find another donor who could be a match for Lisa. Now, kidney paired exchange enables would-be donors like Susan to donate on behalf of a friend; in this process, their kidney goes to someone else whose donor wasn't a match for them, but was for someone like Lisa. These prospective donors decided that they wanted to be part of a KPE program. In Lisa's case a match was found through the National Kidney Registry (NKR), and the transplant date was scheduled.

A few weeks before the scheduled transplant, however, Lisa became sick. Illness can cause a change in one's immune system that in turn can impair compatibility. A repeat cross-match showed that Lisa could no longer get a transplant from the donor at Hospital A as planned. This was again shattering news for Lisa, who was getting sicker.

I found it really hard to be the one to tell Lisa that she could not get her transplant. In nursing school they tell us that as a professional you should not get emotionally involved with your patients. This is impossible for me working so closely with recipients and donors. I cried with Lisa and her mother that day and worried that Lisa might have to start dialysis soon.

Susan wanted her friend to get a transplant, so she decided to proceed with the donation to the recipient at Hospital B, which would give Lisa the chance to receive a living kidney transplant later after she had recovered from her illness. Susan went on to donate on the original date. This is called *advanced donation* and allows the recipient to be transplanted when he or she is medically cleared to proceed.

Lisa recovered from her illness, but her kidney failure symptoms were getting worse. She was waking up every morning nauseated and swollen. This is common when kidneys are failing and is a sign that the patient should start dialysis. Lisa was in her doctor's office discussing starting dialysis when I called her to let her know I'd just learned that a living donor had been found for her through the kidney registry. She had a successful transplant and is now back to work. She told me recently that she has not felt this good in many years.

Bill and Don

Sometimes a person's decision to donate leads to unexpected dramatic benefits for the donor as well as the recipient, in the form of a healthier lifestyle.

Bill was born with polycystic kidney disease, which is hereditary. His kidney function was declining, and he was close to starting dialysis. Recently he had gone to a family reunion and met a cousin whom he had not seen in many years. After the reunion they started to talk more often, and Bill confided that he needed a kidney transplant.

Don immediately talked with his wife about the possibility of donating his kidney to Bill, and after doing research he decided that he would like to do it. Don came to our center in San Diego for the medical testing. During the testing, Don learned that his blood sugar readings were higher than what was acceptable for a kidney donor. He clearly had not expected to be told he could not donate. He was very upset and resolved to change his eating habits and start exercising to improve his blood sugars.

Don met with the dietitian at the transplant office, and together they prepared a plan to help him lose weight. He changed his diet to include fewer carbohydrates, completely stopped eating sugar, and started exercising daily. Don was determined to help his cousin, so he made it his mission for six months to make changes that would help him reach his goal of donating his kidney. He traveled back to San Diego about six months later for retesting. He had lost more than twenty-five pounds and his lab testing had improved; Don no longer was prediabetic. He was approved for kidney donation, and a month later he successfully donated to his cousin Bill.

Ramiro and Diana

The even-longer waits for a kidney for certain recipients can be debilitating and exasperating. Ramiro and Diana had been married for fifteen years and had three children when Ramiro was diagnosed with kidney failure, due to diabetes, and started dialysis. Diana had hoped that she would be able to donate her kidney to him, but she was a blood type A and Ramiro was type O. Their only options were KPE or a deceased-donor transplant. In San Diego the average waiting time for an O recipient on the deceased-donor waiting list is eight to ten years. In a KPE program, however, finding a match in this situation can take one to two years on average.

Ramiro and Diana entered the KPE program as their best option. Ramiro called me every few months, frustrated that he had not yet gotten a transplant offer. I explained that there are not enough O donors, who can donate to any blood type, in the KPE program and that I would call him as soon as he received an offer. He was discouraged and even angry at times, but all I could do was assure him that the waiting time was less in the KPE program and urge him to stay positive.

After Ramiro had been waiting for more than five hundred days, a match was found for him. I was relieved and happy for both him and his wife. The cross-match was done, and he was compatible.

Ramiro and Diana came in for pre-surgery labs and to see the surgeon. During this visit, they discovered that Ramiro had an infection, which meant he could not have the scheduled transplant. The nondirected donor could not wait for Ramiro to recover, so the transplant had to be cancelled. Naturally, Ramiro and Diana were shattered. He had waited so long for a transplant and now it seemed to be out of his reach once again.

About an hour later I got a call from Diana. She wanted to know if she could still donate on the same day to the recipient in the KPE. She said she did not want another recipient to have to experience what her husband was feeling. She explained that she had already scheduled the time off work and that Ramiro would be there for her during her recovery. I was amazed and impressed that Diana was able to have such compassion for someone she had never met. She proceeded with the donation, and Ramiro and her children were at her bedside during the recovery.

Once Ramiro's infection was cleared, I reactivated him in the KPE. About two months after the original transplant date, Ramiro was successfully transplanted, and the new kidney worked immediately.

Steve and John

Often kidney disease is silent and is not diagnosed until someone has an accident or is seen for a routine physical. That is what happened to Steve. He fell and broke his arm, went to the emergency room, and was told he needed surgery. When he had blood drawn in preparation for the surgery, it showed that he was in kidney failure. He was in shock! How could he have kidney failure when he was able to do his normal activities and did not even feel sick? That's why we say it's often silent: no symptoms.

Healthy kidneys filter out toxins and keep the electrolytes in our body balanced. With failing kidneys, Steve's potassium level was critically high, and if left untreated could have led to his heart stopping. He had to start dialysis immediately. Then he was referred for kidney transplant.

Initially Steve had identified a few friends who could possibly become living donors. We started testing to determine whether they were compatible. Steve recently had been in contact with his half-brother, John. They had not had much contact over the years, mainly because they lived in different states. When John found out that Steve needed a kidney, though, he did not hesitate to be tested. John was the best match among the donors who were tested. He completed the donor evaluation and was approved for living kidney donation.

The surgery was scheduled for April. A few weeks before the scheduled surgery, Steve got sick. He had been doing peritoneal dialysis and had gotten an infection, peritonitis. The transplant had to be postponed. Steve had to have the peritoneal tube removed and started temporary hemodialysis. Once the infection was cleared, the surgery was rescheduled for August.

A few days before the rescheduled surgery, John got the flu. Again, the surgery had to be postponed. Steve felt as if he was on a roller coaster. Twice he thought he was going to get a transplant and get back to feeling better.

Fortunately, he kept a positive attitude through it all. I explained that once John recovered, we would reschedule the transplant.

The surgery was rescheduled for September. Steve, John, and I all counted the days until the transplant. The day before the transplant, I checked in with both of them. They were feeling well, and I kept my fingers crossed that the third time would be the charm.

I'm happy to say that Steve had a successful transplant, and his kidney is still working well many years later.

Latisha and David

Sometimes donation circumstances have an added layer of complexity. Latisha was in her early thirties when she came to the transplant center and had known since she was ten years old that she would eventually need a kidney transplant. She had been diagnosed with a kidney disease that causes the kidneys to fail over time. Kidney transplant is the best treatment option for kidney failure, so it was important to identify her living donor before her kidneys completely failed. She was referred to the transplant center before she needed dialysis. Her cousin David had offered to donate his kidney to her. David's father, who had died a few years earlier, had always said that when Latisha needed the transplant, he would be her donor. David remembered this and wanted to do what his father could not.

David was from another country; to donate a kidney, he would need to get a visa to travel to the United States. The transplant center is ready to write letters for the donor requesting a visa to give to the US Embassy, but this does not always result in the donor's being approved for the visa. Happily, David was granted a visa. He was able to come to San Diego and successfully donated to his cousin Latisha a short time later.

West Coast Donor, East Coast Recipient

Up until very recently, living donors always had to have the donation surgery in the same hospital as the transplant recipient. When a donor lives far from the recipient's transplant center, it may be difficult for the donor to travel to a distant city and be away from his or her family and work. That's why one such West Coast donor, Jan, contacted me last year and said that she wanted to donate to her friend on the East Coast but that it would be impossible for her to travel that far to donate. She was responsible for her elderly mother's care and could not be gone for the amount of time required for recovery.

I reached out to NKR and the transplant center to see if they would be willing to help facilitate Jan's request. The donation was performed at our center several months later, and NKR was able to successfully transport Jan's kidney to her friend on the East Coast. The transplant was a success.

This exciting effort initiated the practice of *remote kidney donation* with a direct donor; the system enables someone to donate a kidney to the intended recipient in a distant city without requiring the donor to travel there. It utilizes proven logistics systems, pioneered by NKR in kidney swaps over the past decade, to safely transport the kidney to the recipient's transplant center even if it's thousands of miles away. I would love to see more centers get involved in this.

I always try to treat each living donor and recipient as I would treat my own family. I hope that I can provide information and support that helps to make the process less stressful for them.

Note: The National Kidney Registry is the largest of several donor exchange programs in the United States and accounts for 70% of all U.S. paired donations. Established in 2008, it has the biggest living kidney donor pool in the world and uses computer technology to find the best matches for recipients, leading to better outcomes.

CHAPTER 22

Researcher as Caregiver

by Sharon Williams

Sharon Williams is an associate professor at the University of North Carolina at Chapel Hill whose research focuses on caregiving of people with chronic illnesses.

FOUR YEARS INTO OUR MARRIAGE, we got the news that my husband's kidneys were failing (he was only thirty-seven and I was thirty-four). While words like creatinine, phosphorus, and potassium would soon become part of our lives, at the time all we knew was that Larry's kidneys were failing.

Of course, kidney disease affects the entire family (spouse, children, extended family). My academic research focuses on families who provide care for older adults with chronic illnesses. Conducting this research gives me insight into how family members can have an impact on adjustment to a disease and also on management of a chronic disease. However, in my personal role as the wife of a man with end-stage kidney disease, I learned that though knowing might help the intellectual part of caregiving, that knowledge does not necessarily help the emotional component of family caregiving.

We all handle stress, crisis, and illnesses differently. For many people, a big stressor is being unable or unwilling to accept and respect another's rights to handle a serious illness in his or her own way. That was certainly true for me. When we first found out about Larry's kidney disease, I immediately went into research mode. Did you know that if you eliminate meat from your diet, you can take a big workload off the kidneys and that you may be able to postpone dialysis? I was immediately ready to eliminate meat from our diets. Of course, we would also need to drastically decrease salt—also no bananas, no sodas, on and on. I did not realize at first that I was moving forward based on what I would have done if I were the person who had received the diagnosis of kidney disease. However, I came to realize that I needed to step back and give Larry the space to take the lead on how to handle his diagnosis.

As I now think back, I would likely have been more helpful to Larry if I had just hugged him, told him how sorry I was that he had to deal with this problem, and assured him that we were in it together. I truly think it would have been better to ask him if he wanted me to research possible ways to delay dialysis. That way, he would have been more likely to buy into the findings. I was trying to be the best helpmate I could be, but from the perspective of what I thought best, rather than seeking to understand from him how I could be the helpmate he most needed.

Along the journey, I learned to accept and respect that my husband, a smart and reasonable person, was capable of making decisions related to his health. If he preferred steak, pork chops, and other meats rather than a life without meat, I needed to accept that and not see it as an affront to me, or a lesser way of handling the diagnosis. If he preferred Carolina Treet barbeque sauce (even after I pointed out its astronomical sodium content) rather than a barbeque sauce with lower sodium, it was a choice made by a smart and capable person. I needed to find a way to respect his choices. After all, Carolina Treet was the barbecue sauce his mother used and perhaps the taste of it felt like a safe landing for him in the midst of turmoil.

In the beginning stages of learning to accept and respect Larry's choices, yet also ensuring that more kidney-friendly choices were available, I nagged and took it personally when his choices were not "what I would have done." Two important things: (1) Nobody wants a wife who nags—the Bible says it is better to live on the corner of a roof than to share a house with a nagging wife (Proverbs 21:9 HCSB); (2) Nagging was bad for my emotional health and it in no way supported Larry. I had to learn to accept and respect his ability to make his own choices.

When Larry started dialysis, with some help from me and his doctors, he chose peritoneal dialysis, which exchanges fluids through a tube in the abdomen. Learning to view the catheter as a part of his body and incorporating it into the most intimate parts of our lives took some time. It became our new norm, but it did take some adjustment. Finding a location to store all those boxes that are delivered to your house, incorporating the exchanges into your daily life and into travel—it all was an adjustment. When we traveled, I would usually sneak away from activities to sit with Larry while he did his exchanges. In hindsight, I wish I had made time to sit with him even more often during his exchanges. It would have been a private time for the two of us to share in "this new thing" that had become a part of our lives.

Over the course of several years and several infections, Larry needed to transition to hemodialysis, done at a center using a machine. That felt huge. Nobody wants to do any type of dialysis—however, to move to having to go to a dialysis unit three times a week for half a day was another period of major adjustment.

Larry had a big personality and a beautiful bass voice, and he was friendly. This helped tremendously in his interactions with the nursing staff, the front desk staff, and other people receiving dialysis. He particularly liked Hazel, an older woman who also received dialysis. He made several other good friends in the unit: people he checked on when they were not feeling well and people who checked on him. The need to get to dialysis three times a week can be restrictive; it can also be challenging. During bad weather and poor travel conditions, individuals still need dialysis. Yes, it can be challenging and it can be restrictive, but as with many things, it becomes a part of life, not the entirety of life.

Given the Medicare and Social Security benefits that came along with the diagnosis of end-stage kidney disease, and the disability pay and retirement funds from his job, Larry opted for disability retirement. Considering that Larry did not feel well and was probably depressed when this decision was made, we did not discuss it much. It just seemed like the logical step to take.

Being on disability retirement did eliminate a lot of responsibility, but it also left Larry with much unstructured time. Fortunately, he was able to use his beautiful bass voice to pursue his love of singing. He wrote and recorded some songs, and structured his time around his love of music. However, in hindsight, pursuing the possibility of some time off from work, and perhaps a different role within his work site, might have been better for him emotionally and for his identity as a worker and provider. I came to realize during this journey how much of our identities we often link to our work.

Navigating healthcare is complicated. Understanding the forms and the processes during a time when you are emotionally reeling is difficult. This is something that I hope healthcare providers and coordinators will understand and remember. I also hope people in hospital cafeterias and other support staff will understand and remember that patients and families visiting hospitals and clinics may be emotionally fragile. Once, in the hospital cafeteria, when I was trying to order a salad, a worker became frustrated with how long it was taking me to make a choice. Tears fell from my eyes; ordinarily her frustration would not have made me cry—but I had a sick husband and at that moment, it was just too much. I know she felt bad, but her attitude was just more than I could handle. Another time, when Larry was hospitalized in the ICU and physically suffering, hearing the nursing staff talking and laughing outside his room felt very disrespectful. I know they have lives too, but I encourage healthcare providers to remember that there are people nearby who may be very emotionally and physically fragile.

Again, I encourage you as a spouse or partner to offer your support—that is, help, but do not take over. Consider how much of the time you spend talking with the doctor during medical appointments versus the amount of time your spouse spends talking. Continue trying to understand how you can best support your spouse. Also, consider that your spouse most likely needs private time with his or her doctor without you in the room.

Yes, as a spouse you are indeed affected by this entry of kidney disease into your lives. During the first rounds of Larry's medical appointments, a social worker turned to me and asked, "How is this affecting you?" I cried; it was the first time anyone had asked about the effects of all of this on me. It may also have been the first time I actually acknowledged how this change in our lives had affected me. I think it is important that you remember to take care of your own emotional and physical health.

This arrival of kidney disease—it is tough and it affects the entire family. However, it can provide opportunities to advocate, and it can also increase your compassion for others. I often said, "I have a PhD and it's complicated for me"—what about individuals with poor literacy skills? My aunt would often remind us of how fortunate we were that we had resources that allowed me to take time off from work and accompany Larry on many of his doctor's appointments. That was indeed true, and I often wondered about spouses who had few or no sick days; about who was available to look after their children while they went to doctor appointments; about the high cost of hospital food, the cost of parking, etc. Walking through this journey with Larry increased my understanding of how challenging it is to navigate healthcare and it increased my compassion for others.

There will undoubtedly be family, friends, and others who ask how they can help. As much as you can, be specific with them. Think about it, talk it over with your spouse, and when people ask, have something to tell them. Our family, friends, church members, co-workers, and our dog, Rusty, were invaluable resources. They helped us so much, and they stood with us during the long journey of Larry's illness.

Larry was valiant and he was indeed a kind person, and a good husband. He died on December 19, 2012, after a nineteen-year journey through kidney disease, subsequent liver disease, and a liver-kidney transplant that worked for twelve years.

I knew that making end-of-life decisions and coping with death were tough. But I knew it intellectually. Grief has weight; yes, it can feel like a physical weight that you carry with you—I didn't know that until Larry died. You realize that your head knows that your loved one has died, but it takes your heart longer to know—I learned that too after Larry died.

I knew that I needed to walk through my pain and I knew that I needed to cry my tears. Therefore, I joined a support group, I prayed, and I asked others to pray for me. When people asked how I was doing, I let them know when I was struggling. It's been the most difficult challenge I have ever faced, but a co-worker told me, one day the good memories will override the memories of suffering. She was right: my memories today are not weighed down by the suffering, and my appreciation of life and my compassion for others are heightened.

When I look back, and think about the best suggestion I can offer, it comes back to supporting your partner without taking over. No matter how much you want to help, or manage, ultimately you are not the person with the disease. I encourage you to walk through the journey with your loved one and to be the helpmate that he or she needs you to be.

CHAPTER 23

How a Would-Be Donor
Became an Advocate

by Jenine Lewis

*Jenine Lewis is a volunteer donation advocate through Donate Life/WELD
San Diego.*

YOU DON'T HAVE TO BE a living donor to promote living donation. Despite all
the best intentions and firm commitment, not everyone who wants to be a living donor can be one. I tried my best to donate my kidney to a good friend—
and got *very* close—but ultimately the donation system worked as it should
and prevented me from doing something that could have jeopardized my own
health. I learned how to better protect my kidneys and also learned that there
are many other ways to encourage living donation and to help people who
need a kidney.

I've always been interested in living donation. As a child with a diabetic
sister, I wondered if Gail would someday need one of my kidneys. Fortunately,
she never did. As an adult, I registered as a bone marrow donor, although I was
never called to donate.

A few years ago I met Sharon, a sweet woman with polycystic kidney
disease, which causes clusters of cysts to form in the kidneys. A normal kidney
is the size of your fist and weighs about five ounces. Sharon's kidneys were the
size of footballs: each one weighed fifteen pounds. The cysts in her kidneys
often burst, sending infected pus into her bloodstream and urinary tract. Over
time the cysts would cause renal failure and she would need a transplant. I

wasn't surprised to get an email in July 2015 that Sharon sent to her friends. She was in end-stage renal failure and needed a kidney. Immediately I knew I wanted to be her donor, but I was a fifty-nine-year-old grandmother with a few health problems of my own. Still, I decided to pursue being a donor because I knew I would regret it if I didn't try.

My husband, Alan, thought I was nuts, but I initially allayed his fears by assuring him that I would not commit without his agreement. I then called the phone number listed in the email, connecting me to the transplant coordinator at the center. She told me that Sharon would not be told that I was being evaluated and that I could stop the process at any time for any reason. That impressed me and further reassured my husband. As it turned out, I was the only one of Sharon's friends who was being evaluated as a donor.

After some initial testing to see if I was a good candidate for donation, I was scheduled for two days of thorough testing at the transplant hospital. All of my medical costs were paid for by Sharon's insurance. Potential donors do not pay any medical costs. This was the most comprehensive physical of my life! I had my own team of doctors and nurses, separate from Sharon's so there would be no external pressure on me to donate. My team did not even know who Sharon was. Their focus was on how a kidney donation would affect my health.

The comprehensive physical revealed some problems that I needed to address over the next several months. I never knew that NSAIDs (non-steroidal anti-inflammatory drugs) for pain relief were hard on kidneys, and I had been taking one of them, Advil, for years for my migraines. As a result, I was told my kidney function was lower than it should be. They said I was a borderline donor, and that if I stopped taking Advil, I could be approved as a donor. My husband came with me to meet the surgeon, and having the opportunity to ask several questions about the recovery and what my quality of life would be like as a donor was instrumental in reassuring both of us. Alan gave me his blessing, and I was ready to move forward!

During the next two months, I tried alternative medications and lifestyle changes to treat my migraines, which helped a little. In the meantime, Sharon learned that her surgery would be complicated, because her giant polycystic kidneys needed to be removed, and the donor kidney transplanted. Consequently, she was referred to a surgeon at a different transplant center in another state and asked me if I would be willing to start the process all over again at the new center. Of course, I said yes. I wanted Sharon to have the best surgeon for her situation. In July 2016 the new transplant center approved me to be a donor but also cautioned that I was considered borderline because of my kidney function. A date was set in October 2016 for our surgeries.

I felt nervous about being a "borderline donor." What would that mean for both Sharon and me? Was I making a wise decision for my own health? Would Sharon rather have a different kidney? Sharon and I talked about it. She assured me that she was happy to have my kidney. I asked her to send out an email to her friends, telling them I was approved as a donor but that I was borderline and to please pray for us. We also posted on Facebook about our upcoming surgeries. As we learned later, this was a smart thing to do because it stirred the heart of her friend Alane to consider being a kidney donor.

October came, and Sharon and I traveled to the transplant center with our husbands. There was much excitement. Photos were taken and posted on Facebook. We had our bags packed for our hospital stay. Typically, a donor will spend two or three nights in the hospital, so I had my new pajamas, along with books and magazines to read during my stay. After fifteen long months, with many hurdles to jump, Sharon and I eagerly awaited the transplant surgery that would take place the next morning. We showed up at the hospital for some final routine blood tests. I met with my surgeon, who initialed the skin over my right kidney with a Sharpie. Sharon and I named it Sidney the kidney. We went back to the hotel in the early afternoon.

I then received a call from the nephrologist assigned to me. After reviewing everything, including the results from the blood test I had that morning, she would have the final word on whether I could donate. The doctor was concerned about my kidney function being a little lower than when I had been evaluated three months earlier, and she requested I come back to the hospital for more extensive tests. I nervously did the testing and went back to the hotel. Sharon and I talked about the last-minute preparations. (We assumed the doctor was just being cautious and really didn't think it would be a problem.) Our husbands were going to drive us to the hospital early the next morning for the transplant! In a few hours, it would be over.

While we were eating dinner, the nephrologist called again. "Mrs. Lewis, I am sorry to tell you that your kidney function has fallen below what we consider to be a safe level for you to donate." She explained how my life would be negatively affected if I were to donate and why the surgery therefore had to be cancelled. She patiently gave me all the time I needed for questions. My kidney function had been just under the acceptable level a few months before, she said, and a different nephrologist had assumed that it would not go down—and might even go up—because I'd stopped taking NSAIDs. I was very angry and upset at the time of the phone call. Today, though, I greatly admire the doctor who cancelled the surgery: it took courage for her to do it.

I burst into tears as soon as I hung up the phone. What would I say to Sharon? Would it take another fifteen months for her to get another donor? How could we have come so far and have it be cancelled? I felt like a failure.

Sharon and I talked about it with our husbands and we prayed and we cried. That evening, the night of the cancelled surgery, we decided to send out emails and post on Facebook about what had happened. This was emotionally difficult to do. But many people were following our story. Perhaps someone would come forward to donate.

Remember Alane, Sharon's friend who a few weeks earlier felt that she could be a donor? When she heard that our surgeries were cancelled, Alane contacted Sharon and told her that she would like to be evaluated to be her donor! In addition, three other people who had been following our story by email and Facebook contacted Sharon to donate their kidneys! This was such good news. As it turned out, Alane was a great match for Sharon, and her kidney had a much higher function than mine. Their transplant operations took place only a few weeks after mine was cancelled because the hospital, unusually, had fast-tracked the donor evaluation process in view of the setback. Both donor and recipient are doing well.

I have no regrets about trying to be a donor. There were so many positives that happened. I got the best physical a person can get, and I know a lot more about my body. I learned how to improve my kidney health, which had suffered from those years of taking Advil for migraine headaches.

In the end, the system worked as it should. Transplant centers take the health of their donors *very* seriously. They will not let people donate, as much as they may want to, if it will damage their health or put them at any risk. A prospective donor can back out anytime, for any reason, even minutes before the surgery. Similarly, the doctors can call a halt to the process at any point if they have concerns, as in my case.

It was helpful that Sharon shared her story publicly on Facebook, and by sending out emails. This was hard for my shy friend to do, but it clearly made a difference, and moved just the right person to want to be a donor (and a few others). There is hope for those who need a kidney and great rewards for those who donate, or who try to donate as I did!

And I found a wonderful alternative way to help even more kidney patients, donors, and other borderline donors: as a volunteer with WELD (Women Encouraging Living Donation), a nonprofit group based in San Diego. We get the word out through billboards and by speaking at service clubs, showing up at charity race events in our WELD tee shirts to cheer on racers, and having one-on-one conversations about living donation. Sometimes I console disappointed would-be donors, like me, and encourage them to advocate for their loved ones through social media.

The time and effort are definitely worth it when I see the smiles of the recipients—and the donors! I can personally attest that you don't need to be a living donor to promote living donation.

What's on the Horizon?

For Living Kidney Donation and Transplantation

WE'VE ALREADY SEEN THE LANDSCAPE change dramatically from the days not so long ago, when Carol donated her kidney (2006) and Betsy had her transplant (2004). Back then, kidney exchanges weren't even a blip on our radar; even less so were voucher programs to enable someone to donate now and give a loved one a voucher for a kidney down the road. Nonmilitary drones weren't even in use then, and now they're transporting kidneys from someone who's just died, avoiding inner-city traffic when every minute outside the body reduces its chance of success, to a waiting recipient. And organs that used to be discarded as unusable, or simply undesirable, are now being readily and gratefully accepted: for example, through the HOPE Act, HIV-positive kidneys are successfully being transplanted into HIV-positive patients, and the practice has recently been expanded to other organs, mainly livers.

For most of us, this was all unthinkable just a few short years ago.

That should give us hope that today's seemingly futuristic headlines about enhanced robotics and other promising developments may also see the light of day in the next decade. Example: transplanting organs from genetically engineered pigs. Apparently, pig kidneys are incredibly similar to human kidneys on a cellular level and hold the most promise for use in humans.

Most exciting of all the dramatic prospects on the horizon is a small, surgically implantable, permanent, bio-artificial kidney. Because it doesn't involve the immune system, there would be no need for antirejection medications, with their accompanying drawbacks. And even well-matched living-donor kidney transplants don't last forever, so *permanent* is indeed an exciting prospect.

The bio-artificial kidney has been in development at the University of California at San Francisco since 2015. Initial clinical trials for "the Kidney Project" have been pushed back repeatedly. In the best of times, this was always a very ambitious project, and then it ran into 2020. Predictably, progress slowed substantially because of COVID-19 and funding needs. At this writing, the Kidney Project tentatively plans to start the trials sometime in 2021.

These are all very promising efforts, but some aspects of these innovations will take many years to perfect. And even if all the exciting developments could dramatically cut the waiting list in half, the wait for a kidney for most people would still be too long. There will still be heartbreaking stories such as the Facebook post a few years back "written by" a six-month-old baby whose mother had been on dialysis for six hours a day, six days a week while pregnant. The young mother had become blind from diabetic retinopathy and couldn't even see her new baby. Fortunately, the dramatic post, which was the grandmother's idea, was a success: a stranger, a young mother of six, donated one of her kidneys.

So for now, kidney patients and families: if conventional methods for finding a living donor haven't worked, keep trying novel ways, with Facebook posts, podcasts, tweets, cruising billboards, or whatever. But we all need to continue to push state legislatures and Congress to find ways to increase organ-donor registration with common-sense measures, and to provide protections and supports for living donors. The Living Donor Protection Act will be reintroduced in 2021, in the 117th Congress, but it's just a start. Let's keep the pressure on the lawmakers to pass this and other important measures like increased funding for financial assistance for donors and scientific research on long-term ramifications of living donation and research on better treatments for chronic kidney disease and, ultimately, a cure.

If living donors like Carol and thousands of others can manage to convey to potential donors that unbeatable sense of satisfaction that comes from giving a piece of yourself to enable another human being to live a fuller life, we will be that much closer to eliminating the kidney shortage and saving many more lives.

For Betsy

When Betsy's kidney transplant reached the fifteen-year mark, she began to have health issues that indicated she would need another transplant. After notifying family, friends, and colleagues, and encouraging them to spread the word, she found a donor, Tiffany Woynaroski. The transplant surgery was scheduled, but just weeks before the surgery Betsy began having problems with her liver, which is also polycystic, so the transplant was cancelled. She was later told she would need both a kidney and a liver transplant. She was on the UNOS list for both organs and had dialysis four times a week at home while continuing her work as a professor.

On May 26, 2021, Betsy got "the call" and received a kidney and liver transplant from a deceased donor. (FYI: Her first donor, Linda, is fine.)

For Carol

Carol continues to enjoy excellent health and an active lifestyle. Her 0.75 creatinine reading would be enviable for any nondonor of her age or younger. Her surgery scars have faded to the point of invisibility, but her gratification and interest in living donation have only grown with the years. (FYI: Despite some earlier challenges, Paul is doing well after nearly fifteen years with Carol's kidney and looks forward to many more with it.)

Frequently Asked Questions

Contents

Potential Donors

How might COVID-19 affect my ability to donate a kidney?

Whether or not you have been exposed to someone with COVID-19, it is likely that as part of the screening process, and later before the transplant, you will be given one or more lab tests to determine whether you have COVID or have been exposed to it. The results of the tests will determine the next steps in the process. If either the donor or recipient has COVID-19, a transplant cannot take place until both people test negatively for the virus and have undergone a quarantine period.

If I have had COVID, can I donate my kidney?

Having had COVID does not exclude you from donating a kidney. The transplant team will let you know when you will be free from infection, and you may have to postpone the surgery. Be sure to discuss this with the transplant team.

Will I be more at-risk of getting COVID after I donate a kidney?

At this time there is no evidence that donating a kidney puts you at higher risk for getting COVID. As with all donors following donor surgery (or any surgery), taking time to recover before resuming normal activity is advised.

Is it safe for living kidney donors to get a COVID-19 vaccine?

Currently, living donors are considered part of the general public and thus can safely take the vaccine. Guidelines for the general public are subject to change as information continues to emerge on the safety and effectiveness of the vaccines. It's always best to consult your healthcare provider about your individual situation. The American Society of Transplantation (AST) posts updates to a fact sheet about the vaccines: https://www.myast.org/

Who pays for my donor testing and the surgery?

Your recipient's health insurance will typically pay for all the testing and donation surgery costs, whether it's private health insurance or Medicare. Medicaid usually does as well, but in exceptional cases, your costs may not be covered in some states. It is essential to verify this information because it can change from year to year. Also, in all cases, routine tests such as Pap smear or colonoscopy would be your own (or your health plan's) responsibility.

Who pays for any additional expenses I might incur as a donor?

"Incidental expenses" are not included in the recipient's health insurance coverage of donor costs under most plans, so any additional expenses for transportation and lodging for an out-of-town stay, lost pay, or possible childcare costs are your own responsibility. Fortunately, financial aid is increasingly available. Donation-related medical/prescription costs after leaving the hospital are usually covered, but your own health insurance could be used if they are not. The donor social worker and the financial coordinator at the transplant center can provide details on diverse sources of donation-related financial assistance. (See the Appendix for a list of such organizations and sources of information on fundraising strategies.)

If my donor evaluation discovers a possible medical condition, who pays for any additional tests?

If the condition would need to be treated whether or not you donated, your own insurance plan would be responsible for the tests and any treatment needed.

How safe is live-kidney-donor surgery?

The risk of surgery-related death for a donor nephrectomy (kidney removal) is extremely low, about 3 in 10,000, which is typical of many major surgeries. Similarly, there is an associated risk of infection, bleeding, and hernia.

What happens if I have donor surgery–related complications at a later date?

If the complications occur during the two years following the donation, the transplant center is usually responsible for providing care to the donor. Beyond that period, the situation varies not only by center but also depending on the medical condition and the recipient's and donor's health insurance.[21] This is something a potential donor should try to clarify with the center.

Are there any long-term health risks for living kidney donors?

Although rare, the main risks concern a slight increase in blood pressure and in the chance of someday developing kidney failure; the *actual* lifetime risk of kidney failure is still extremely low, however, about 1%. A major study reported in *JAMA: The Journal of the American Medical Association* in 2014, which followed every living kidney donor in the United States (96,000+) for up to fifteen years after donation,[22] concluded that compared with similarly healthy individuals who did not donate, kidney donors had "a somewhat higher estimated risk of developing ESRD" (about 1%) but still a much lower risk than the general population (about 3%).

What happens if I later develop kidney failure after donating and eventually need a transplant?

In the exceedingly rare event (less than 1%) that you later needed a transplant, you would be given very high priority on the kidney waiting lists, assuming you were a good surgery candidate. UNOS, the nonprofit organization that manages the lists for the federal government, places prior living donors in a category just below children but ahead of the majority of adults on the kidney-alone waiting list. The list also assigns points for various factors, so instead of a typical years-long wait for a deceased-donor kidney, as a previous living donor you would mostly likely receive a kidney in a few months. And if you donated through the National Kidney Registry, it similarly grants priority to previous donors, so you might have a living donor within weeks or months.

Are there any future pregnancy concerns for living donors?

Most centers now advise female donors to wait a year after the surgery before becoming pregnant; some also advise waiting a year after giving birth *before* donating. The majority of kidney donors who later become pregnant have uncomplicated pregnancies, but some studies have found an elevated risk of gestational hypertension and preeclampsia, which can sometimes lead to dangerously high blood pressure and protein in the urine. Although the probability for the most serious outcomes "remains low," you should definitely raise any relevant concerns during your donor evaluation.

What would be a typical timeline for my donor testing and surgery?

The timeframe for the entire process will vary depending on scheduling constraints, availability, and your possible need for any follow-up testing. Medical tests, appointments with a psychologist, a social worker, financial counselor, a transplant nephrologist, and a transplant surgeon—and, of course, the wait for surgery—usually take anywhere from one to six months. When time is critical, some centers allow donors to check into the hospital for the testing or have it all done on two consecutive days.

Are there specific requirements concerning a donor's weight?

Many transplant centers use a body mass index (BMI) cut-off for eligibility because obesity increases the chances of developing diabetes and hypertension, the major risk factors for kidney disease. A BMI of 30 or higher indicates obesity, but cut-offs for donating vary considerably by center, anywhere from 30 to 40 BMI. Many centers will offer you consultation with a nutritionist if you need to lose weight and advise you on how to do so in a healthful way.

Are there age restrictions on being a living kidney donor?

Many centers prefer that donors be 65 or younger, although most have no strict upper age limit; a donor's overall health and the kidney's health matter the most. (We know donors who were in their mid-70s when they donated.) Like Carol, a third of living donors are over 50 and their numbers are increasing. However, there is less chance that an older person will be able to pass the necessary medical tests to ensure that donation would be safe for both the recipient and the donor.

Most centers have a *minimum* age of 18, but many consider that too young to make such a life-changing decision and often prefer that a donor be over 25. Even then, given the need for more long-term studies of donor risks, many experts are reluctant to encourage people in their twenties to make non-directed donations because it is not known whether they are likely to develop kidney disease themselves.

If my local transplant center rejects me as a kidney donor, could I apply at another center?

Yes. Even though some conditions are universally recognized as unsafe for donation, such as diabetes and uncontrolled high blood pressure, acceptance decisions on other issues can vary from center to center.

What happens if I change my mind about donating once I've started the evaluation?

You need never worry that you cannot change your mind. Up until and including the very day of the surgery, you will be asked to confirm your decision. If you decide not to go ahead with the donation, your reasons will remain confidential unless you choose to discuss them.

Could an adult donate a kidney to a child?

Yes. Although it is not a given that even a parent will be a match, it is not uncommon for a parent to donate to his or her child—even a toddler. An adult-size kidney can often fit inside a young child's body and will provide more kidney function than a healthy child-sized kidney.

How many days will I need to stay in the hospital after my donation?

For a routine laparoscopic nephrectomy, which is now done in 99% of cases, you should expect to stay in the hospital for just one to two days. An open nephrectomy, which requires a slightly larger incision and potentially more pain, could entail a stay of three to five days.

How much pain should I expect after donating and how is it managed?

The most significant pain usually occurs in the first two or three days, often at the incision site and in the shoulders and collar bones (oddly, it arises from the gas used to inflate the abdomen during surgery). Because most transplant centers have tried to reduce opioid use, some centers have eliminated or reduced donors' use of the push-button pain medication pump. Instead, they give injections at the incision site during surgery and pain medications before, during, and after surgery; some perform a nerve block on the abdominal wall that lasts about twenty-four hours.

You'll be urged to walk a bit the same evening. The movement is critical to relieve the gas pain and to help prevent pneumonia and intestinal blockage. You'll probably graduate to oral pain meds before leaving the hospital. Many donors also find that an elastic abdominal binder or a pillow helps reduce pain.

About how long should my recovery take as a donor?

It takes about six weeks to get back to full energy level and resume most activities but only a matter of days before your body starts the renewal process. You will probably want to take it easy for the first few days after leaving the hospital but are encouraged to take walks and even to go up and down the stairs at home as needed if you feel up to it.

The day after Carol came home, she took a ten-minute walk and made the walk a bit longer or faster each day after that. She continued to enjoy an afternoon nap for a few weeks.

How soon could I go back to work after donor surgery?

If you have a sedentary job, you might be ready to resume a reduced schedule in about two weeks, depending on whether the job entails driving. Driving is usually permitted after two weeks but is a function of pain at the incision site and use of pain medication. Because of a prohibition against lifting objects weighing more than ten pounds for at least six weeks, if you are a laborer or someone whose job entails heavy lifting, you may be told to wait two to three months to resume work.

If I do not have enough sick leave to cover the time I need to take off work, as a living donor, will my job be protected by the Family and Medical Leave Act (FMLA)?

Yes. Since 2018 employers are required to grant FMLA protections to living donors. Also, the proposed federal Living Donor Protection Act would provide additional protections (some states have already enacted their own versions). Some donors, like Carol, use short-term disability insurance or have access to a shared-leave program that allows coworkers to donate leave to an employee in need.

Will I have any dietary restrictions after donating?

Any dietary constraints are typically in the first week or so following surgery and involve the need to ensure regular bowel movements, which are usually sluggish after major surgeries, particularly with the use of painkillers. You will be advised to eat fruits, vegetables, and fiber and to stay hydrated. Beyond the initial period, you'll simply be encouraged to eat a healthy diet and to drink plenty of fluids. There are no protein restrictions, but avoid protein shakes or powders.

Will I have any constraints concerning medications after donating?

You will be advised to eliminate or minimize the use of NSAIDs (nonsteroidal anti-inflammatory drugs, like ibuprofen), which can cause acute kidney injury. Some centers provide a list of other medications to be avoided. When prescribed new medications, it is always wise to remind your provider or pharmacist that you have only one kidney and to consider any potential for kidney damage. For example, IV antibiotics are permissible, but the physician may need to alter the dosage because of your having only one kidney. You should not need to take any kidney-related medications.

I've always been very physically active. Will being a living donor affect my lifestyle?

You should be able to resume the level of activity and lifestyle you had before the surgery. Running, biking, and most physical activities are encouraged—while keeping hydrated—but you will be cautioned against engaging in contact sports or extreme sports because of the risk of injury to your remaining kidney.

What impact will the kidney removal have on my kidney function?

Your remaining kidney gradually enlarges and takes on some of the function of the other kidney. After a few months, your kidney function will reach and stay at about 65% to 75% of pre-donation function, which is sufficient to lead a normal life.

What kind of long-term monitoring will I need to do for my health?

The only ongoing monitoring needed is having your blood pressure and kidney function checked annually, the latter with a simple blood test for creatinine to measure the level of waste products in the blood. This can be done through your primary care provider. Transplant centers are required to follow their living donors for two years post-donation. These follow-ups include blood and urine tests to measure kidney function and look for protein in the urine as well as checking blood pressure and weight, and answering questions regarding the donor's overall health and function.

Will I have trouble obtaining health or life insurance because of being a donor?

For health insurance, the Affordable Care Act protects people with preexisting conditions from being denied or charged higher rates for health insurance. It is certainly in both donors' and recipients' best interests that these protections be safeguarded in any new healthcare plans. For life insurance, sometimes donors can encounter difficulty with some insurers. Your transplant center will typically support your efforts to obtain coverage. It is wise to check on coverage before making the donation. The proposed Living Donor Protection Act provides donors with protections regarding insurance[23] coverage and premiums.

Are there any medical tests I should avoid after donation?

Certain tests such as MRI and CT scans usually entail the use of contrast dyes, which should be avoided if possible—for transplant recipients as well—because they are processed through the kidney. Always tell the prescribing physician and technician that you have only one kidney. If contrast dye is necessary, they can limit the amount used and may give you IV fluids or hydration beforehand.

How soon after my donation can I have sex?

That's purely a personal decision that depends on when you feel ready: typically, between two and four weeks.

How soon can I have a beer or other alcoholic drink after donating?

There are no donor-related restrictions other than with the use of painkillers.

Patients Weighing Dialysis versus Transplant

How might COVID-19 affect my dialysis?

If you receive dialysis at a center and have or are suspected of having COVID-19 and are not severely ill or hospitalized, you will likely be sent to a specialized dialysis unit for just such a situation. You will have dialysis at that center until you have passed the requirements to return to your usual center—for example, no sign of infection, no fever or other symptoms, fourteen-day quarantine following diagnosis or suspicion.

How might COVID-19 affect the possibility of my receiving a transplant?

Whether or not you have been exposed to someone with COVID-19, it is likely that as part of the screening process, and later before the transplant, you and your donor will be given one or more blood tests to determine whether one of you has COVID or has been exposed to it. The outcome of the tests will determine the next steps in the process. If either the donor or recipient has COVID-19, a transplant cannot take place until both people test negatively for the virus and they have undergone a quarantine period.

What kinds of dialysis are there and what is involved for each?

There are two types of dialysis, *hemodialysis* and *peritoneal dialysis*, but patients currently have a few major options: center-based hemodialysis, day or night; home hemodialysis; and peritoneal dialysis (performed at home, center, or workplace). Each method has its benefits and challenges, so patients should be sure to read about and discuss the options with their healthcare team to decide what might be best suited to their health and personal preferences. Failing kidneys have difficulty processing fluid and removing it from the body, so whatever the type of dialysis, excess fluid is drawn out while the blood is being cleaned.

Hemodialysis uses a *dialyzer* to clean the blood outside of the body. An arteriovenous (AV) fistula or AV tube is surgically created under the skin to join a vein and an artery to allow blood to be drawn in and taken out. If done at a center during the day, patients usually start with four-hour treatment times including fifteen minutes on each end for connecting to and disconnecting from the machinery. If done at home, most patients perform it four or five days per week for three hours at a time. In **nocturnal hemodialysis** patients spend usually three nights a week at a dialysis center to have treatment while they sleep; treatment time averages six to eight hours because this dialysis has a slower rate of toxin removal.

Peritoneal dialysis is the most common form of home dialysis. Instead of a machine, it uses the lining of the patient's abdomen (through a network of tiny blood vessels) to filter the blood. A catheter (or tube) is surgically inserted in the abdomen, and through it a cleaning solution is drawn in and then removed. Patients can choose between two types: (1) the patients hang a bag above them, with tubing connected to a catheter to exchange fluid four times a day for about thirty minutes each time; or (2) a machine is attached to the catheter and pumps the fluid in and out of the person's body overnight while they sleep.

Can I live longer if I get a transplant rather than undergo dialysis?

Yes. The five-year survival rate for patients on dialysis is a little more than a third. Given that a deceased-donor kidney functions for ten to fifteen years on average, and a living donor kidney fifteen to twenty years, a transplant typically offers a longer and healthier life than dialysis.

What kinds of differences in my quality of life can I expect after a transplant versus being on dialysis?

Most transplant recipients feel better and have a far better quality of life after a transplant than when they were on dialysis. They also regain independence and time each week now that they do not do dialysis—and no longer need to plan travel around dialysis. However, transplant recipients must seek medical advice quickly for any evidence of illness. Because of needing to take immunosuppressant (antirejection) drugs, recipients are more vulnerable to infections.

What kind of solid and liquid diet would I have to follow on dialysis?

To help make the dialysis process as effective as possible, restricting fluids is very important. Too much fluid can also cause shortness of breath. Salt absorbs water, so keeping a low-salt diet helps reduce the amount of liquid to be removed during dialysis. Salt can cause swelling in the joints, legs, and feet. Most renal diets also encourage reducing the amount of protein, potassium, and phosphorus in food intake. Protein (especially meat) makes the kidneys work harder; therefore, using nonmeat protein such as eggs, cheese, or fish can help. Regulating the amount of potassium is also important, because potassium levels can affect heart rhythms and may cause nausea, weakness, or numbness. Too much phosphorus, as in soft drinks, can also build up, causing the bones to release calcium, leaving them brittle and weak, and can also damage major organs. (See the Appendix for websites with diet and nutrition information sources.)

What are some of the risks in staying on dialysis?

Although dialysis can be lifesaving, being on it for an extended time poses health risks such as anemia, heart or bone disease, infections, and damage to nerves. Further, some patients experience cramping, nausea, weakness, and sometimes depression because of the many restrictions on their lifestyle.

What are some of the risks of transplantation for the recipient?

Transplantation has few risks beyond those posed by any type of abdominal surgery. Most patients (some say 95%) do not have any major complications. The most common complications are the transplanted kidney's not functioning properly or being rejected by the body. Both situations are fairly rare. Also, the vast majority of transplant recipients must take antirejection drugs for the rest of their life; these medications can make you more susceptible to infections and add a small risk of cancer.

Does a transplant cost more than staying on dialysis?

No. In fact, a transplant is actually less expensive than long-term dialysis. Some sources indicate that a transplant can cost between $100,000 and $250,000, whereas the cost of dialysis is about $90,000 per year. The cost to you as the patient will vary by the type of insurance you have and whether you have Medicare. Talk to a transplant clinic financial counselor to find out approximate costs given your own circumstances.

Could I get a transplant without being on dialysis?

Yes. For example, if your kidney function is declining rapidly and you already have an identified donor, you can discuss with your physician the possibility of doing a *preemptive transplant,* that is, a transplant before you need dialysis. Patients who can avoid dialysis typically have more successful long-term transplants.

Potential Transplant Recipients

How might COVID-19 affect the possibility of receiving a transplant?

Whether or not you have been exposed to someone with COVID-19, it is likely that as part of the screening process and later before the transplant you and your recipient will be given one or more lab tests to determine if you have COVID or been exposed to it. The outcome of the tests will determine the next steps in the process. If either the donor or recipient has COVID-19, a transplant cannot take place until both people test negatively (i.e., they don't have the virus) and they have undergone a quarantine period.

If I or my donor have had COVID, will we still be able to complete the transplant?

Your transplant team will tell you when you are both clear of infection and it is safe to complete the transplant.

Am I more likely to get COVID after a transplant?

Because of needing to take immunosuppressant drugs after transplant, you will be considered high risk and will need to take extra precautions to not be exposed to others who may have COVID. Because you are high risk, you may be at increased risk of getting any disease or having a more severe case of COVID if you get it.

If I don't have a living donor and I'm on the waiting list for a deceased donor, what are the most important factors that will decide whether I get an available kidney?

Although there are many complex considerations, for the average adult, how long the person has been waiting is still the major factor in getting a kidney offer. Therefore, it is very important to be evaluated by a transplant program when your kidney function is just over 20% so you can start to gain "waiting time" on the list once your function reaches 20% or lower. If you take good care of yourself, you may be able to have several years before your kidney function declines enough to require dialysis (and might even be able to receive a deceased donor transplant before starting dialysis).

UNOS (United Network for Organ Sharing) is the private, not-for-profit entity under contract to run the federal Organ Procurement and Transplant Network and manage the national waiting lists for deceased-donor organs; OPTN oversees the clinical aspects. OPTN/UNOS considers a combination of blood-type and antibody matching, amount of time with kidney failure, medical urgency, likelihood that the kidney will survive, proximity to the donor location, and a few other factors[24] such as being a child or being a previous live kidney donor. In recent years, *longevity matching,* or how closely a recipient matches the age of the donor, is also considered. Candidates who best meet the combination of factors receive the highest priority.

What other factors are considered in the allocation of kidneys to people on the waitlists?

The *Estimated Post Transplant Survival (EPTS)* score (0% to 100%) is assigned to all adult candidates on the kidney waiting list and is based on four factors: time on dialysis, current diabetes diagnosis, prior solid organ transplants, and candidate age. Further, the wait time on the transplant list now includes either when the person began dialysis or was placed on the waiting list and when his or her GFR dropped below 20.

What are the medical options for recipients who have incompatible living donors?

Recipients who cannot receive a kidney from their potential donor—in some cases, from *any* donor—now have a few other options. In nearly all instances, participating in a kidney paired donation (see section *Both Donors and Transplant Recipients,* later in the FAQs) and receiving a biologically acceptable kidney is the safest option. In addition, two kinds of programs are available at some transplant centers:

Blood Type Incompatible Donors

To receive a kidney from a donor with an incompatible blood type, recipients are given five to ten *plasmapheresis* treatments before and sometimes after the transplant. A process similar to dialysis, plasmapheresis removes harmful antibodies that can cause the patient's body to reject the donor's kidney. Some patients also have their spleens removed at the time of surgery to lower the number of cells that produce antibodies.

Positive Cross-match and Sensitized Patient Kidney Transplant

A similar program makes a transplant possible for a patient whose donor may be blood-type compatible but who has developed antibodies against that donor—known as a *positive cross-match*. These patients may receive strong medications to decrease their antibody levels, may undergo plasmapheresis treatments to remove the harmful antibodies from their blood, or both. If and when their antibody levels are reduced, they can proceed with having the transplant.

Can I be listed for a kidney transplant at more than one transplant center?

Yes. Most patients choose to be on the list of the closest center (there are about 250 in all), but being listed in centers that are far apart might boost your chances of getting an organ. The downside to multiple listings is that you may need to complete some required testing for each center (however, most tests may be transferable), and being closer to home for follow-up visits can save money and time. Talk with your nephrologist about these options and make sure each center allows multiple listings.

Can I transfer my time on a transplant waiting list from one center to another?

Yes, the time you have spent on a center's list should transfer to a new site. However, be sure to double-check that the new center will accept your waiting time from the first center. This is an advantage only if you were listed before you started dialysis. Otherwise, your waiting time anywhere will be from the start of your dialysis.

How long do most transplanted kidneys last?

The *average* life of a transplanted live-donor kidney generally has been cited as fifteen to twenty years, but many recipients have had their transplants for more than thirty-five years. Most kidneys transplanted from a deceased donor do not have as long a lifespan; the average is ten to fifteen years, and more than thirty years is very rare.

Will having a transplant increase my life expectancy?

Yes. U.S. kidney patients will usually live twice as many years post-transplant as they would if they had stayed on dialysis. Recent improvements in both surgical techniques and antirejection drugs have resulted in longer life expectancies for both deceased-donor and live-donor kidney transplants.

How many days will I have to stay in the hospital for a transplant?

You will likely stay in the hospital for three to five days after your transplant, assuming no complications. If your kidney is slower to start, you may stay seven to ten days.

What happens during my hospital stay after the transplant?

The healthcare team will continually monitor your urine output and blood pressure, generally every hour for the first day, and then usually every six hours over the next few days to make sure there are no signs that your body is rejecting the new kidney or evidence of other blood chemistry issues. You generally will have blood tests right after surgery and then every morning. You will be started on two or sometimes three antirejection medications and may be provided physical therapy to help you get back to normal movement. A transplant nurse coordinator will work with you during your hospital stay to educate you about medications, home care, any physiological issues, and to set up follow-up appointments with your healthcare professionals after discharge.

What happens in the weeks post transplant?

You will need to stay within easy driving distance of the hospital or a local lab for a few weeks so the team can monitor the new kidney's function, perform blood tests at least weekly, manage medications, and monitor your overall health. Most labs can perform the tests you need, and your healthcare team can help confirm this. In the early days, you will have more frequent visits and blood work. You will also need to check your blood pressure and body weight daily in the beginning to make sure they stay steady; once they do, you can monitor them a little less often. The transplant team will give you detailed information about whom to call if you have any concerns, and someone from the team will be on call 24/7, for both emergencies and questions.

How long is a typical recovery time for a transplant recipient?

Your recovery could take anywhere from eight to twelve weeks as you gradually return to normal activities. However, if your health before surgery was particularly poor (or there were complications after surgery), that may extend the recovery time. You probably won't be cleared by your doctor to drive for four to six weeks, because of any pain medications you might be taking, and also to make sure your surgical incision is healing well.

How soon can I go back to work after my transplant?

You will most likely be back to work after eight to twelve weeks, although you might gradually begin working part-time before then, depending on the physical demands of your job. The more active the job, the more recovery time needed. If you have to park far from your work site, you may initially want to have someone drive you to and from work. In case your employer is not very flexible, or if you have limited sick leave, be sure to ask your transplant team to write a letter *before* the surgery indicating why it would be helpful for you to have a Family and Medical Leave, which can provide up to twelve weeks of unpaid, job-protected leave per year.

How much pain should I expect from the transplant and how is it managed?

The pain that results from a kidney transplant is typical of most abdominal surgeries and will vary from person to person. As with most surgeries, the first few days will be the hardest, and it is important for your healthcare team to develop a good pain management plan. If it isn't taking care of most of your pain, be sure to let them know. Some surgeons actually begin some type of pain medication at the site of the incision just before finishing the surgery, in addition to the general anesthesia administered.

How is pain medication administered following transplant surgery?

For the first day or two, you may have a PCA (*patient-controlled analgesia*) medication pump connected to your IV so that you can administer the pain medicine when you need it. Don't worry about getting too much, because the pump allows only a certain number of doses each hour. Before you leave the hospital, the team will transition you to oral pain medication. You are likely to need the pain medication the first week following surgery, with lessening amounts over time. Gradually, you can move to over-the-counter pain medications such as acetaminophen and soon reduce its use.

Does the pain medication have side effects?

Yes—the most common side effect is a slowing of the intestinal system from both the abdominal surgery and the pain medication; most providers will advise you to take stool softeners at the same time. Also, some people get sick to their stomach or itch from certain pain medications. Be sure to alert your doctor or nurse if side effects appear so that other medications can be tried or additional ones administered to reduce these effects.

What types of other medications will I need after a transplant?

Soon after the transplant, you will be started on a range of medications. The most important are antirejection drugs such as cyclosporine or tacrolimus, mycophenolate, and prednisone (a steroid that may be excluded from the regimen for certain patients). These medications are critical in suppressing your body's natural tendency to attack a foreign body—your new kidney—which usually protects us. In addition, for the first several months you will probably be put on anti-infection medications such as Bactrim (or Septra) and Valcyte, to prevent "opportunistic infections" in your lungs and viral infections; antihypertension medications such as atenolol or metoprolol if needed; stool softeners; calcium; magnesium; and any medications for cardiac function or lipid lowering—plus other medications you may have been taking before the transplant, unrelated to kidney disease.

How many medications should I expect to take following a transplant?

In the beginning, you will take quite a few at least twice a day. You may easily take twenty to thirty pills a day at the start as the medication helps your body get accustomed to the new kidney. Over time, the doses may be adjusted and some medications stopped. This fluctuation in medication is typical following a transplant and will eventually stabilize with only occasional modifications needed later. Except in extremely rare cases, you will need to stay on antirejection medications for the rest of your life.

What side effects from the transplant medications should I be on the lookout for?

You should be aware of small changes in your body and in how you feel: appetite, digestion, energy level, bowel habits, fluid retention, mood changes. Note particularly any changes that may be signs of infection, such as pain, fever, vomiting, or urinary problems like burning, frequent urination, or blood in your urine. Significant changes that last more than a few days should be brought to the attention of your medical team.

One of the side effects that Betsy experienced was related to the steroids: the base of her tongue and cheeks became enlarged and began to block her airway when she was sleeping. She went to an ENT (ear, nose, and throat doctor) because she began snoring, woke up feeling that she had hardly slept, and was falling asleep during the day. A sleep study confirmed that she had sleep apnea, and Betsy received a continuous positive air pressure (C-PAP) machine; after a few days of using the C-PAP while she slept, her energy level returned to normal, and now she sleeps comfortably with no snoring.

What if the antirejection drugs are incompatible with my other medications?

A number of medications (and foods like grapefruit) are incompatible with some antirejection medications. The transplant team will make sure that all medications you take, both before and after the transplant, are compatible and will not harm your kidney. When seeing nontransplant providers, however, be sure to mention the transplant and your current medications, especially if new medications are being prescribed. Also, check with your doctor before trying any over-the-counter or herbal treatments, because they could interfere with one or more of your medications. Your pharmacist should also provide you with an alert if any incompatible medication is prescribed.

How restrictive will my diet be if I have a transplant?

Your after-transplant diet will not be nearly as restrictive as your diet was if you were on dialysis. If you have high blood pressure, watching salt intake will always be important. Hydration is also important, and some professionals recommend drinking 64 to 80 ounces of liquids per day. Most transplant patients have to give up grapefruit because it interferes with some antirejection medications. Many transplant center websites recommend healthy diet guidelines for kidney transplant recipients, such as getting enough fiber daily and eating lean meats, poultry, and fish.

Are there any restrictions on vaccinations I can have after a transplant?

Avoid all live vaccines, such as measles, mumps, rubella (MMR), and the varicella (chickenpox) vaccines.

Avoid the nasal influenza vaccine (have an injection instead). Flu shots can be given without live virus, so request that version.

Flu shots, for patients who have not received one before transplant, are now recommended right after transplant, followed by a three-month booster.

Get Hepatitis B vaccine before transplant.

Is it safe for kidney transplant recipients to take the COVID-19 vaccines?

Yes. And most health authorities consider that the benefits of the vaccines, which are not live, far outweigh any potential risks. However, the extent of the vaccines' effectiveness for transplant recipients and other immunocompromised individuals continues to be studied. Guidelines for the general public and kidney transplant recipients in particular are subject to change as information continues to emerge on the safety and effectiveness of the vaccines. It's always best to consult your transplant team or healthcare provider about your individual situation. Also, check the National Kidney Foundation's page on COVID-19 vaccines (https://www.kidney.org/) or The American Society of Transplantation (AST) COVID-19 Vaccine Fact Sheet at https://www.myast.org/

If I have an arteriovenous (AV) fistula that was used for dialysis, when can it be removed?

Because recipients sometimes have to return to dialysis if their new kidney begins to fail, some physicians do not recommend removing a functioning fistula, and many recipients share this reluctance. However, an AV fistula poses risks such as bleeding, infection, or nerve injury. Other reasons for closing or removing an AV fistula include risk of heart failure, fistula complications, or cosmetic concerns by the patient. This is a decision that you and your transplant surgeon or nephrologist should make together.

As a transplant recipient, would it be okay for me to swim in a public pool or lake?

Although different transplant teams give differing advice, particularly in the first six months after a transplant, many centers do not restrict their patients on where they can swim. Some suggest showering with antibacterial soap after swimming. Check with your transplant team.

Can I still eat at restaurant buffets after my transplant?

Note: During the COVID-19 epidemic, all buffets were prohibited and it is unknown at this time whether that will be an option once the pandemic has ended. Before COVID, for the first three months, some transplant centers urged patients not to eat at a public buffet. However, restaurant buffets follow certain standards of food preparation and protection, such as overhangs over the buffet and a requirement to get a new plate for each visit to the buffet, so after the first few months, you may not have to worry about eating at some of your favorite spots.

What about sexual relations after my transplant?

Doctors often recommend that you wait between four and six weeks to have sexual intercourse following a transplant. This will give you time to recover from the surgery, have minimal to no pain, and regain some of the stamina you had pre-transplant. Some medications can alter sexual desire, so you may want to consult your doctor if this is an issue for you.

Donors and Transplant Recipients: Paired Donation

What are donor pairs or kidney swaps?

Officially known as kidney paired donation (KPD) or kidney paired exchange (KPE), donor pairs are an increasingly common way to shorten the wait for a lifesaving kidney. The practice enables a kidney patient whose potential live donor is healthy, but not a good match for the patient, to receive a kidney from another live donor who, similarly, is not a match for his or her own intended recipient. Sometimes, several pairs of donors are involved—often in different parts of the country—and these situations are called dominos or donor chains. A donor chain starts with a nondirected donor (a kidney donor who is making a selfless gesture to an unknown recipient). See the Appendix for sources of more detailed information on paired donation.

In paired donation, what is a typical wait time for a kidney?

Depending on all the participants' availability and scheduling, paired donations usually take place within a few months.

Who pays for the donor's costs?

As in any living-donor transplant, the recipient's insurance—whether private insurance, Medicare, or Medicaid—pays for the donor's medical costs. Sometimes the transplant center pays for the donor testing.

Do nondirected donors and recipients always meet each other?

No. That is an individual decision. The transplant center will offer to send a note from one to the other, and it is up to the individuals whether they want to meet or even respond.

What is advanced donation?

Sometimes used interchangeably with a *voucher program*, this recent option allows a donation and a transplant to be separated by months or even many years. A person can donate to a recipient who may be in imminent need before another pairing takes place. The donor's *intended* recipient, who may not yet (or ever) need a transplant, receives a voucher for a future match through the program.

My friend in Oregon wants to donate to me but I'm in Maryland, and she can't travel here. Is it conceivable for her to donate in Oregon?

It may be possible, but not all transplant centers participate in this type of remote donation, so check with your center. The National Kidney Registry, for example, facilitates remote donations in addition to paired donations. Your donor's surgery may in fact be able to be done locally in Oregon and the kidney shipped to your transplant center in Maryland.

Appendix: Resources

I. General Resources

Don't be misled by a name: all or most of the following organizations provide information and services for both potential living donors and patients.

American Association of Kidney Patients (AAKP): Information on kidney disease, resources, advocacy, programs and events, policy and legislation. https://aakp.org/

American Foundation for Donation and Transplantation (AFDT): Association of transplant professionals. Operates Living Organ Donor Network (LODN), a free database so medical professionals can collect individuals' demographic and medical characteristics, store their donor decision, and track their quality of life after donation. Offers insurance for post-donation medical complications. http://amfdt.org/lodn_info.aspx

American Kidney Fund (AKF): Prevention, health education resources, listing of clinical trials, updates on legislation, and financial assistance for patients (including those on dialysis). http://www.kidneyfund.org

American Society of Transplantation (AST): Offers **Live Donor Toolkit:** Resources for Those Considering Live Donation; patient resources (transplant living, oral health, pediatric transplant information, how to apply for National Living Donor Assistance, nonprofit sources of financial assistance); some materials in Spanish. https://www.myast.org/ (main website) http://www.livedonortoolkit.com/

American Transplant Foundation (ATF): Provides educational, emotional, and financial support for living donors, patients, and their families. Can request a free mentor. Information for patients on finding a donor. https://www.americantransplantfoundation.org/

Donate Life America: Living donation, organ donation registry, print and video materials. Has state representatives and provides contact information for those individuals. https://www.donatelife.net/

Donate Life/WELD (WoMen Encouraging Living Donation): Volunteer outreach program connecting potential donors with members; provides home visits and speakers to give presentations. Original San Diego–based all-women group was offshoot of the John Brockington Organization; now has chapters in other states and is affiliated with Donate Life.

Home Dialysis Central: Information on all dialysis treatment options. https://homedialysis.org/

Kidneys In Common. Supports living kidney donation through community building, awareness, and kidney donor support. https://www.kidneysincommon.org/

National Kidney Donation Organization (NKDO; formerly Donor to Donor): Dedicated to helping end the U.S. kidney crisis by educating and supporting prospective living donors. https://www.nkdo.org/

National Kidney Foundation (NKF): Information about donation, family and patient resources, fundraising help, offsetting patients' and donors' out-of-pocket costs (including prescriptions), kidney walks and events, policy and legislation, free health-check locations, peer-to-peer support for donors and recipients, nutrition, recipes, and meals. https://www.kidney.org

Fundación Nacional del Riñón (NKF, Spanish website): http://informate.org/

National Kidney Registry: Largest U.S. paired-donation registry, for people in need of a kidney, considering donation, or interested in a voucher program (allows donors to donate kidney in an exchange before their intended recipient may need it). Its Donor Shield program offers several protections, including financial reimbursement and legal representation, for people who donate through NKR or at affiliated transplant centers. https://www.kidneyregistry.org/

Organdonor.gov: U.S. Government information on all aspects of organ donation and transplantation. Sixteen languages represented. https://www.organdonor.gov/

Organ Procurement and Transplantation Network (OPTN): Data arm for UNOS, information on policy, legislation, data on number of transplants, donors, and resources for patients and professionals. Also has various calculators for estimating post-donation life. https://optn.transplant.hrsa.gov/learn/about-donation/

Polycystic Kidney Foundation (PKD): Dedicated to finding treatments and a cure for PKD, peer mentoring program, online discussions. https://pkdcure.org

Renewal: Orthodox Jewish charity providing information and resources for both donors and recipients, regardless of religious affiliation. https://www.renewal.org

Scientific Registry of Transplant Recipients (SRTR): Guide to Transplant Programs that provides wait times and other center specifics, provides statistical and analytic support to OPTN. http://www.srtr.org/transplant-centers/

Transplant Recipients International Organization (TRIO): International organization with 25 U.S. and international chapters, providing information, communication guides, United Airlines travel program, student scholarships, legislative updates. https://www.trioweb.org

United Network for Organ Sharing (UNOS): Nonprofit organization contracting with federal government to manage the national organ allocation system, matching deceased donors with recipients. Information about kidney transplantation, paired (living) kidney donations, signing up to donate. https://www.unos.org

Waitlist Zero: Policy and donor advocacy, public awareness, and transplant education. For those seeking a donor, advice on informing others about donation. http://waitlistzero.org/

II. By Topic *(sites listed above are cross-referenced here)*

Diet and Nutrition

American Kidney Fund *(see listing above in General Resources).*

National Kidney Foundation *(see listing above in General Resources).*

Financial Assistance *(asterisk denotes services specifically for living donors)*

*American Living Organ Donor Fund: Dedicated to ways to protect living donors from medical and financial hardships. http://www.helplivingdonorssavelives.org/

*American Society of Transplantation *(see listing above in General Resources).*

American Transplant Foundation *(see listing above in General Resources).*

*Donor Care Network: Some donors may be eligible for reimbursement of lost wages, travel and lodging reimbursement, life and disability insurance, and legal representation. Works with twelve transplant centers across U.S. so donors can get testing closer to home if needed. https://www.donorcarenet.org/

John Brockington Foundation: Financial and resource support in San Diego area for donors and recipients; promotes health education to minority communities. http://www.johnbrockingtonfoundation.org

Living Kidney Donor Network (LKDN): Annotated list of organizations that provide financial assistance to recipients and donors. http://www.lkdn.org/financial-assistance

Medicare Prescription Drug Plan "Extra Help": Help with prescriptions through the Social Security Administration. Apply online, https://www.ssa.gov/benefits/medicare/, or visit your local Social Security office.

National Foundation for Transplants (NFT): Fundraising help. http://www.transplants.org/

National Kidney Foundation *(see listing above in General Resources).*

National Kidney Registry *(see listing above in General Resources).*

*National Living Donor Assistance Center: Financial assistance to living donors for out-of-pocket expenses for travel and lodging (based on recipient's income eligibility); expanding assistance to cover lost pay, childcare, and eldercare; and to extend to more donors. https://www.livingdonorassistance.org/

Prescription Assistance. Prescription assistance programs at some drug companies for their medications to those who qualify. https://www.kidney.org/patients/resources

*Renewal *(see listing above in General Resources).*

State Kidney Programs: Offering assistance for kidney transplant or dialysis patients with outpatient medications and other expenses; available in approximately fifteen states.

State Pharmaceutical Assistance Programs: Offered in many states and the U.S. Virgin Islands to help pay drug plan premiums and/or other drug costs.

Medical Advances

The Kidney Project: "Frequently Asked Questions by Patients." University of California at San Francisco's national research project to create a surgically implanted bioartificial kidney. Currently in preclinical trials; timeline further delayed by COVID-19. https://pharm.ucsf.edu/kidney/device/faq and on Facebook: https://www.facebook.com/ArtificialKidney

Online Communities and Blogs

To join a "private" Facebook group, simply search for its page in Facebook, and hit "Join Group." You'll be asked just a few questions.

Could You Be a Kidney Donor? What to Expect If You Give the Greatest Gift: Carol's own website and blog with timely posts on donation- and transplant-related topics, focused on assisting potential living donors. https://www.kidneydonorhelp.com/blog

Kidney Support: Dialysis, Transplants, Donors and Recipients: Private Facebook group with 25,000 members.

Kidney Transplant Recipients & Donors: Private Facebook group with 7,000+ members.

Living Donors Online (LDO): Online community for living donors, potential donors, their families, and medical professionals. http://livingdonorsonline.org/about-us/

Living Kidney Donors Support Group: Private Facebook group with 6,000+ members.

Living with Polycystic Kidney Disease Support Group: Private Facebook group with 9,000+ members.

Top 30 Kidney Donor Blogs, Websites, and Influencers: https://blog.feedspot.com/kidney_donor_blogs/

Transplant Café: Online community and social networking site for anyone involved in transplantation or donation, whether personally or professionally. https://www.transplantcafe.com/

Paired Kidney Donation

Alliance for Paired Kidney Donation (APKD): Detailed information about paired kidney donation, computer algorithm for identifying potential matches, and donor protection programs. http://paireddonation.org/about-us/

National Kidney Registry *(see listing above in General Resources).*

United Network for Organ Sharing (UNOS) *(see listing above in General Resources).*

Search for a Living Donor

American Transplant Foundation *(see listing above in General Resources).*

Living Kidney Donors Network: Information for donors and recipients. Includes webinar, *Having Your Donor Find YOU*, and other information for finding a donor. Contacts for coaching and mentoring. http://www.lkdn.org/

Living Kidney Donor Search: For both potential donors and donor searchers: information and stories. https://www.livingkidneydonorsearch.com

MatchingDonors: Matching services for people in need of various organ transplants (most commonly kidney or liver), including paired kidney donation, https://matchingdonors.com/life/

National Kidney Foundation: The Big Ask, The Big Give: Information on how to start "the conversation"; videos of donors and recipients talking about their experiences. https://www.kidney.org/transplantation/livingdonors

Renewal *(see listing above in General Resources).*

Transportation Services

Air Care Alliance: Volunteer pilots who fly patients for care. Directory of groups by U.S. location. http://www.aircarealliance.org/

American Organ Transplant Association (AOTA): Free ground transportation for patients through Greyhound Bus to and from transplant centers. Request submitted by transplant center. http:/www.aotaonline.org/

Angel Med Flight: Medical flight information for transplant centers (costs usually covered by insurance), information on multiple wait lists, and pre- and post-transplant. http://www.txmultilisting.com/wait.htm

Glossary

ABO blood group system. Also called *blood typing.* System of blood groups that includes A, B, AB, and O blood types. The Rh factor (+ and –) does not matter in an organ transplant.

advanced donation program (ADP). A type of kidney paired exchange, separated in time by months or years. A donor chooses to donate before the intended recipient will have—or even need—the transplant, in the hope that a matched kidney will be available at the time of need. A voucher system is a form of ADP. See **kidney paired donation.**

altruistic donor. See **nondirected donor.**

antibodies. Specialized cells in the body that can recognize "foreign" organisms entering the body and attack and kill them; they normally act as a protective response against bacteria and viruses but could jeopardize a potential organ donation.

antibody screening. Procedure used to test someone's blood to check the type of red blood cell antibodies present, to make sure that the donor and recipient have compatible antibodies.

antigens. Substances that are foreign to the body, such as diseases, viruses, bacteria; when a potential donor and recipient match six out of six antigens, the match is colloquially referred to as a "perfect match." See **HLA.**

antirejection meds. See **immunosuppressant medications.**

AV fistula. Abbreviation for *arteriovenous fistula.* A connection surgically created under the skin to join an artery and a vein, to allow blood to be drawn in and taken out in hemodialysis.

Berger's disease. See **IgA nephropathy.**

blood plasma. The liquid portion of the blood, which contains red and white blood cells, antibodies, and proteins. Makes up 55% of blood volume.

blood typing. See **ABO blood group system.**

BMI. Abbreviation for *body mass index*. A measure of body fat based on weight and height.

Bright's disease. The broad term that used to designate what would now be called *nephritis*.

catheter. A flexible tube used to insert in the body to put in or take out fluids—for example, dialysis catheter, urinary catheter.

chronic kidney disease (CKD). Also called *chronic kidney failure* or *renal disease*. A condition where kidneys gradually begin to lose function and may progress to the point at which they can no longer effectively filter out wastes and extra fluid.

colonoscopy. Test using a small, flexible scope inserted in the rectum that allows a specialist to look at the inside of the intestines and colon.

C-PAP. Abbreviation for *continuous positive air pressure*. A small machine that pumps pressurized air via flexible tubing into a patient's face mask (over nose and in some models also the mouth) to help keep the airway open, mostly used to treat sleep apnea.

creatinine. A waste product in the bloodstream that is filtered by the kidney and then eliminated in urine. It is a key measurement of kidney function, because when the kidneys are damaged they are less efficient at removing creatinine from the bloodstream; the more creatinine in the blood sample, the lower the kidney function.

cross-matching. A test that mixes a patient's blood with that of a potential donor to see if they are compatible; the test is repeated at different points throughout the donor evaluation.

CT scan. Abbreviation for *computed tomography angiogram*. Series of X-ray images taken from different angles that results in cross-sectional images of the bones, blood vessels, and soft tissues inside the body. In a donor evaluation, the test results help the surgeon decide which kidney to take.

desensitization. A process called immunoglobulin (IVIG) therapy to make the body less sensitive to outside substances by slowly introducing antibodies; sometimes used for patients who have such a sensitive immune system that kidney donation is not possible.

diabetes. A chronic condition that affects the way the body processes sugar, through an inability to produce or respond to the hormone insulin. It is the most common cause of kidney failure in the United States.

dialysis. A treatment that does many of the things a healthy kidney would do to clean a person's blood by removing waste and excess fluid from the body. See also **hemodialysis; peritoneal dialysis.**

donor chain. Also called *domino chain* and initiated by a nondirected donor, who donates to an unknown recipient, leading to multiple sets of transplants. See also **kidney paired donation**.

donor coordinator. A member of a hospital transplant team, usually a registered nurse, who performs intake and arranges testing, interviews, and related activities for donor evaluations, organ donation, and transplantation.

EKG. Abbreviation for *electrocardiogram*. A test that looks at the electrical activity of the heart.

EPO. Abbreviation for *erythropoietin*. A hormone produced by healthy kidneys that prompts bone marrow to make red blood cells.

EPTS. Abbreviation for *estimated post-transplant survival*. A score from 0% to 100% assigned to all adult candidates on the kidney waiting list (for organs from deceased donors), based on four factors: candidate time on dialysis, current diagnosis of diabetes, prior solid organ transplants, and candidate age.

ESRD. Abbreviation for *end-stage renal disease*, the point at which a person's kidney function is too low to sustain life—that is, requiring dialysis or a kidney transplant.

fistula. See **AV fistula**.

FSGS. Abbreviation for *focal segmental glomerulosclerosis*. A rare kidney disease in which scar tissue forms on the parts of the kidneys that filter waste from the blood (glomeruli) and can lead to kidney failure.

gestational hypertension. High blood pressure that develops during pregnancy.

GFR. Abbreviation for *glomerular filtration rate*. Considered the best measure of a person's kidney function (as a percentage of functioning nephrons—filtering units—within the kidney) by considering their creatinine level with their size, age, sex, and race. A GFR under 60 may show kidney disease (less relevant in a living donor); under 20 indicates kidney failure.

glucose tolerance test (GTT). A blood test that measures how well the body processes sugar before and after drinking a syrupy solution; most commonly used to diagnose gestational diabetes but also used as a screening test for Type 2 diabetes.

Good Samaritan donor. See **nondirected donor**.

heart stress test. A test done to determine whether the heart gets enough oxygen and blood flow while a person is exercising. Usually done on a treadmill or stationary bike; when exercise is not possible because of physical limitations, a chemical is injected into the bloodstream to simulate "exercise-induced" stress.

hemodialysis. A type of dialysis that uses a machine to replace kidney function by filtering the blood outside of the body using a dialyzer (artificial kidney); it can be performed at a dialysis center, at a hospital, or at home. It usually approximates 20% of normal kidney function.

hemoglobin A1C (HbA1C or A1C). A test that shows the average level of blood sugar over a roughly three-month period: a common test for diabetes (normal is 4 to 5.6%; diabetes is above 6.5%).

HLA. Abbreviation for *human leukocyte antigen*. A set of six genes that regulate the immune system and make up a person's tissue typing (after blood typing, the other factor in testing compatibility). HLA tests are required before a transplant to check whether the donor's and recipient's tissues match on the six relevant antigens.

hypertension. Abnormally high blood pressure.

IgA nephropathy. Also called *Berger's disease*. A kidney disease caused by an antibody, immunoglobulin A (IgA) entering the kidneys and making them less efficient by damaging their filtering system.

immunosuppressant medications. Also called *antirejection medications*. Drugs that nearly all transplant recipients must take to keep the body's immune system from building up antibodies (that is, that reduce or suppress its strength) so it won't attack the new kidney.

independent living donor advocate (ILDA). An advocate at a transplant center who provides guidance to donors to protect their rights and confirm informed consent; federal regulations require transplant centers to provide an ILDA to all donors.

intravenous (IV) line. A method of injecting liquid medications, fluids, or nutrients directly into a vein.

KDRI. Abbreviation for *kidney donor risk index*. An index that combines a variety of deceased-donor factors into a single number to summarize the risk of a kidney failing after the transplant.

kidney exchange. See **kidney paired donation.**

kidney paired donation (KPD). Also called *kidney paired exchange, kidney exchange,* or *kidney swap.* A way for multiple recipients whose intended donors may not be a match for them to achieve a match by swapping with different donors. When more than two pairs are involved, it is called a donor chain and is initiated by a nondirected donor.

kidney swap. Informal term for *kidney paired donation.*

laparoscopy. A modern, minimally invasive surgical method that uses a tiny lighted tube to guide surgery of the abdominal or pelvic organs; it's the predominant method used for living kidney donation.

living donor. Term referring to a healthy person who donates a kidney or, less commonly, a segment of the liver or lungs.

longevity matching. A process for allocating kidneys to people on the UNOS waitlist so that kidneys expected to last the longest go to people who are expected to live the longest.

mammogram. X-ray pictures of the breasts to look for lumps or other signs of breast cancer.

matching. A process for ensuring that a donor and recipient are a good match for transplantation. Three blood tests are used: blood typing, tissue typing, and cross-matching.

medication pump. See **patient-controlled analgesia (PCA) pump**

MRI. Abbreviation for *magnetic resonance imaging*. A test that uses a magnetic field, radio waves, and a computer to produce images of the organs and structures in the body.

nephrectomy. The surgical removal of a kidney.

nephritis. Also called *glomerulonephritis*. A group of diseases that damage the tiny filters (glomeruli) of the kidneys.

nondirected donor. Formerly called *altruistic donor*; sometimes called *Good Samaritan donor*. A person who donates to an unknown recipient, usually initiating a donor chain. See also **kidney paired donation**.

NSAIDs. Abbreviation for *nonsteroidal anti-inflammatory drugs*. Medications such as ibuprofen used to reduce pain, swelling, and fever.

obesity. An unhealthy excess of body fat (differs from being *overweight*), often defined by a body mass index (BMI) above 30.

Pap smear, Pap test. A routine screening test for women to look for cancerous or precancerous cells on the cervix.

patient controlled analgesia (PCA) pump. A medical device that delivers a patient's pain medication intravenously in response to his or her push-button control; the amount of medication is regulated to prevent overdose.

peritoneal dialysis. A type of dialysis that uses the lining of the patient's abdomen (through a network of tiny blood vessels) to filter the blood, instead of a machine as in hemodialysis; it inputs a cleaning solution into the abdomen and then draws it out. It is similar to hemodialysis in efficiency but is done daily.

peritonitis. An infection of the lining of the patient's abdomen (peritoneum), a common, serious complication for patients receiving peritoneal dialysis.

plasmapheresis. A filtering machine process (similar to dialysis) for removing plasma that may contain antibodies, and replacing the affected plasma with unaffected plasma.

polycystic kidney disease (PKD). A genetic disease that causes fluid-filled cysts to grow in the kidney, which leads to high blood pressure and often to kidney failure.

preeclampsia. A condition that can develop during pregnancy and lead to dangerously high blood pressure and protein in the urine.

psychosocial. Combining psychological factors and social environment.

pulmonary (lung) function test. Sometimes called *spirometry*. A group of noninvasive tests, including spirometry, to determine how well the lungs are working, specifically how well a person is able to breathe in oxygen and breathe out carbon dioxide, and how efficiently the person can get oxygen to the vital organs.

remote donation. A type of living kidney donation in which a donor is not required to travel to the recipient's transplant center for the kidney removal; the donation is performed at the donor's local center and the kidney is safely shipped to the recipient's transplant center.

renal ultrasound. A noninvasive test that uses sound waves to examine the kidneys, ureters, and bladder.

transplant nephrologist. A physician with a specialty in nephrology who works with kidney patients considering a transplant and with potential kidney donors.

transplant nurse coordinator. A member of a hospital's transplant team who manages testing and evaluation, and provides care to a transplant donor or recipient. In most cases, the donor and recipient will have separate transplant nurse coordinators.

transplant psychologist. A psychologist who gathers information from and conducts tests with donors or recipients to make sure they have the emotional and mental health to go through the transplantation or donation process.

transplant social worker. A social worker who gathers information from and often performs psychosocial assessments of donors or recipients; also advises on post-donation and post-transplant financial and social supports.

transplant surgeon. A surgeon who specializes in performing organ transplants and removing donor organs.

transplant team. The team of providers—usually a nurse coordinator, psychologist, social worker, transplant nephrologist, and transplant surgeon, sometimes physician's assistants (PAs)—who work with the donor or recipient to prepare for, perform, and monitor after a donation or transplant.

ultrasound. A noninvasive procedure that uses sound waves to examine bones, blood vessels, and organs within the body.

UNOS. Abbreviation for the *United Network of Organ Sharing*. A nonprofit organization that manages the list of patients in the United States who are in need of transplantation; allocates deceased-donor organs only.

X-ray. A noninvasive imaging procedure, such as a chest X-ray, that can show bones, organs, and blood vessels inside the body.

Notes

Chapter 1: Why We Need More Living Donors

1. Updated references for most of the U.S. transplant facts and figures in this chapter can be found on the following websites: https://www.organdonor.gov/, https://www.donatelife.net/, and http://www.kidneyfund.org/.

2. built-in supports a government creates along with it: Some research suggests that presumed consent alone "is not the magic bullet." More recently, logistical objections and concerns have also been raised. See "Presumed Consent Not Answer to Solving Organ Shortage in U.S.," Healthcare-in-Europe.com.

3. finding a compatible donor for them can be extremely challenging: Desensitization treatments in such cases were considered "revolutionary" in 2016 (Kolata, "Desensitization Treatments") but are rarely used now because other options are considered safer.

4. focus on medical innovation: These efforts built on earlier actions stemming from the 2016 White House Summit, at which a broad group of government agencies, universities, and organizations announced major commitments to reduce the organ shortage. The Summit featured a $160 million public-private investment in "biofabrication" techniques that basically use the principles of 3D printing to repair and replace tissues and cells.

Chapter 2: Before You Make That Call

5. kidney failure is less than 1%: Muzaale et al., "Risk of End-Stage Renal Disease."

6. to discuss their individual risks in detail: You can do a rough calculation of your Living Donor Risk Index by plugging in just a few key characteristics, at http://www.transplantmodels.com/donesrd/.

7. extended multicenter studies of donor risks are certainly needed: The longest-term studies have gone out fifteen to twenty years, at a single center.

8. donors lose some kidney function, the impact is usually not significant: Donors lose 25% to 35% of their pre-donation kidney function, which is still sufficient to live a normal life.

9. living with one kidney has minimal ramifications: Most kidney diseases are systemic, so they typically affect both kidneys at the same time—that is, having one or both kidneys would not make a difference.

10. can then have a healthy pregnancy: see Frequently Asked Questions, "Potential Donors," for information on pregnancy-related concerns.

11. "96% felt it was a positive experience": Najarian, Living Donor Kidney Transplants.

12. long-term health problems following their donation: Unfortunately, there are no national statistics on the frequency of such problems; more long-term studies are critically needed. In 2018, a ten-center pilot program, the Living Donor Collective, began to track living donors' health for the rest of their lives. Neergaard, Push to Better Track Living Kidney Donors' Long-term Health.

13. are surely the most altruistic of all: In her book The Fear Factor, psychologist Abigail Marsh, who studies altruism, terms nondirected donors "extraordinary altruists."

14. finding a kidney for a particular recipient: A national living donor registry is being developed to gauge intent to become a living donor when someone registers as an organ donor. The registry would also provide a way to harness the spike in interest that often follows an individual's well-publicized plea for a kidney.

Chapter 3: The Preliminaries

15. volume of living-donor and deceased-donor transplants: https://optn.transplant.hrsa.gov/data/.

Chapter 5: Tackling Potential Donor Obstacles

16. four times as likely as whites to develop kidney failure: Recent research suggests that a genetic component present in some African Americans may be less important than the prevalence of risk factors such as diabetes and hypertension. "Blacks Face a Higher Risk of Kidney Failure," Science Daily.

17. 1.3 times that of non-Hispanics: These statistics and others on minorities and kidney disease are available on the Donate Life website: https://www.donatelife.net/news/2020.

18. can be a game changer for a lot of people: NLDAC eligibility guidelines can be found on its website, at https://www.livingdonorassistance.org/. NKR's Donor Shield program goes even further, providing various protections that include coverage for some

usually noncovered donation-related medical and related expenses even several years after the donation. The Alliance for Paired Kidney Donation recently added some of these protections for its donors.

19. widespread government reimbursement of related expenses: You can find the official summary and details of the latest federal efforts to remove financial disincentives here: https://tinyurl.com/2b52yj5q.

20. uncomfortable idea of paying for body parts: In Kidney for Sale by Owner, bioethicist Mark Cherry makes a strong case that a well-regulated transplant organ market could save more lives while not exploiting the poor.

Frequently Asked Questions

21. recipient's and donor's health insurance: For people who donate through the National Kidney Registry—or at an affiliated transplant center—the Donor Shield program covers later, usually noncovered, donation-related medical and related expenses. The Alliance for Paired Kidney Donation recently added some of these protections for its donors.

22. for up to fifteen years after donation: An earlier, smaller study of 3,000+ living kidney donors covered a period of twenty to thirty years. It found "no significant difference" on several indicators compared with their nondonor siblings. The study was limited, however, by being done at a single center where nearly all of the patients were white. Najarian, Living Donor Kidney Transplants.

23. provides donors with protections regarding insurance: The proposed Living Donor Protection Act of 2019, which would prohibit insurance companies from discriminating against living donors, among other protections, is expected to be reintroduced in 2021. In the meantime, several states have already enacted or are preparing legislation providing these and other protections.

24. proximity to the donor location, and a few other factors: OPTN is finalizing a major change in the system, which had previously given priority to location. If no eligible candidate can be found within a 250-mile radius, the changes require looking first for the closest but then for the best candidate elsewhere in the country while still giving some priority for proximity. In addition, in December 2020 the Centers for Disease Control and Prevention announced changes to make the allocation system, which has come under increasing criticism for waste and variations in efficiency, more accountable and flexible. For more information on this very complex system, see the Frequently Asked Questions at the UNOS website, https://www.unos.org.

Selected Bibliography and Suggested Reading

In addition to the Appendix resources and the transplant centers and individuals we've consulted, here is a list of some of the publications and resources that have informed our thinking and that may also be of interest to readers.

Books

Cherry, Mark J. *Kidney for Sale by Owner: Human Organs, Transplantation, and the Market*. Washington: Georgetown University Press, 2005.

Marsh, Abigail. *The Fear Factor: How One Emotion Connects Altruists, Psychopaths, and Everyone In-Between*. New York: Basic Books, 2017.

Mezrich, Joshua D. *When Death Becomes Life: Notes from a Transplant Surgeon*. New York: Harper, 2019.

Simon, Risa. *In Pursuit of a Better Life: The Ultimate Guide for Finding Kidney Donors*. Transplant First Academy, 2017.

Sytner, Ari. *The Kidney Donor's Journey: 100 Questions I Asked Before Donating My Kidney*. Ari Sytner, 2016.

Books for Children

Cortez, Brenda E. *Howl Learns About Kidneys and Dialysis*. Mukwonago, WI: Nico 11 Publishing and Design, 2019.

Cortez, Brenda E. *My Mom Is Having Surgery: A Kidney Story*. Mukwonago, WI: Nico 11 Publishing and Design, 2018.

Morsi, Nadine. *Kinsey's Kidney Adventure*. Herndon, VA: Mascot Books, 2017.

Newspaper and Magazine Articles

"Blacks Face a Higher Risk of Kidney Failure Than Whites, Regardless of Genetics." *Science Daily*. March 10, 2016.

"France Introduces Opt-out Policy on Organ Donation." *The Guardian*, Jan. 2, 2017.

Kolata, Gina. "Desensitization Treatments in Preparation for the Transplant: New Procedure Allows Kidney Transplants from Any Donor." *New York Times*, March 9, 2016.

Kragen, Pam. "New Women's Group Encourages Kidney Donation." *San Diego Union Tribune*, Jan. 30, 2017.

Leins, Casey. "Should the Government Decide If You're an Organ Donor?" *US News & World Report*, Feb. 12, 2016.

Neergaard, Lauran. "Push to Better Track Living Kidney Donors' Long-term Health." *Denver Post*, Jan. 29, 2018.

"Pervasive Myths and Misconceptions about Organ Donation Still Exist in the Black Community." *Pittsburgh Courier*, June 25, 2015.

Snowbeck, Christopher. "UnitedHealthcare Will Cover Travel Costs for Kidney Donors." *Star Tribune*, June 13, 2016.

Tonelli, Marcela, and Gill, John. "Our Medicare Policy for Kidney Transplants Is Totally Irrational." *Washington Post*, Dec. 6, 2017.

Vavra, Kassidy. "At 84, Texas Man Is Oldest Living Kidney Donor in U.S." *New York Daily News*, May 31, 2019.

Zickl, Danielle. "Yes, You Can Run an Ultra with 1 Kidney—This Donor Proved It." *Runner's World*, Oct. 17, 2018.

Journal Articles

Cheng, Xingzing S., Glassock, Richard J., Lentine, Krista L., et al. "Donation, Not Disease! A Multiple-Hit Hypothesis on Development of Post-Donation Kidney Disease." *Current Transplantation Reports* 4 (2017): 320–326.

de Vries, Laura, Tent, Hilde, Sanders, Jan-Stephan, et al. "Low GFR after Kidney Donation Is Not Chronic Kidney Disease." *2013 American Transplant Congress*, Abstract number 198.

Gill, John S., Delmonico, Francis, Klarenbach, Scott, and Capron, Alexander M. "Providing Coverage for the Unique Lifelong Health Care Needs of Living Kidney Donors within the Framework of Financial Neutrality." *American Journal of Transplantation* 17 (May 2017): 1176–1181.

Hunt, Heather F., Rodrigue, James R., Dew, Mary A., et al. "Strategies for Increasing Knowledge, Communication, and Access to Living Donor Transplantation: An Evidence Review to Inform Patient Education." *Current Transplantation Reports 4* (March 2018): 27–44.

Jay, Colleen L., Dean, Patrick G., Helmick, Ryan A., and Stegall, Mark D. "Reassessing Preemptive Kidney Transplantation in the United States: Are We Making Progress?" *Transplantation* 100 (May 2016): 1120–1127.

Joshi, Shivam, Joshi, Sheila, and Kupin, Warren. "Reciprocating Living Kidney Donor Generosity: Tax Credits, Health Insurance and an Outcomes Registry." *Clinical Kidney Journal* 9 (Feb. 2016): 168–171.

Kumar, Keertini, Tonascia, James M., Muzaale, Abimereki D., et al. "Racial Differences in Completion of the Living Kidney Donor Evaluation Process." *Clinical Transplantation* (May 23, 2018): e13291.

Lam, Nagan N., Lentine, Krista. L., and Garg, Amit X. "End-Stage Renal Disease Risk in Live Kidney Donors: What Have We Learned from Two Recent Studies?" *Current Opinion in Nephrology and Hypertension* 23 (Nov. 2014): 592–596.

LaPointe Rudow, Diane, and Cohen, David. "Practical Approaches to Mitigating Economic Barriers to Living Kidney Donation for Patients and Programs." *Current Transplantation Reports* 4 (March 2017): 24–31. [Topical Collection on Live Kidney Donation, K. L. Lentine, section editor]

Lentine, Krista L., and Segev, Dorry L. "Understanding and Communicating Medical Risks for Living Kidney Donors: A Matter of Perspective." *Journal of the American Society of Nephrology* 28, no.1 (2017): 12–24.

Najarian, John S. "Living Donor Kidney Transplants: Personal Reflections." *Transplantation Proceedings* 37 (Nov. 2005): 3592–94 (Department of Surgery, Fairview-University Medical Center, Minneapolis).

O'Keeffe, Linda, Ramond, Anna, Oliver-Williams, Clare, et al. "Mid- and Long-Term Health Risks in Living Kidney Donors: A Systematic Review and Meta-Analysis." *Annals of Medicine*, Feb. 20, 2018.

Segev, Dorry L., Muzaale, Abimereki D., Caffo, Brian S., et al. "Perioperative Mortality and Long-term Survival Following Live Kidney Donation." *JAMA: The Journal of the American Medical Association* 303, no. 10 (2010): 959–966.

Serur, David, Pesavento, Todd, Poglio, Emilio, et al. "Life with One Kidney: Primary Care and the Living Kidney Donor." *America Journal of Medicine* 130, no. 7 (2017): 763–765.

Sontrop, Jessica M., and Garg, Amit X. "Considerations for Living Kidney Donation Among Women of Childbearing Age: Evidence from Recent Studies." *Current Transplantation Reports* 3 (March 2016): 10–14.

Van Pilsum Rasmussen, Sarah E., Henderson, Macey, Kahn, Jeffrey, and Segev, Dorry. "Considering Tangible Benefit for Interdependent Donors: Extending a Risk–Benefit Framework in Donor Selection." *American Journal of Transplantation* 17 (Oct. 2017): 2567–2571.

Online Publications and Blogs

Agar, John. "The Mathematics of Dialysis vs. Two Normal Kidneys." Blog post, Dec. 1, 2016. https://tinyurl.com/y82rpqub.

Baker, Talia. "Living Donors and the True Power of Facebook Virality." *Huffington Post* blog, June 9, 2016. Updated June 10, 2017. https://tinyurl.com/ybe8yrqa.

Elflein, John. "Top 10 U.S. hospitals by number of organ transplants performed between 1988 and 2019." *Statista*. Jan. 29, 2020. https://tinyurl.com/u56oo8t.

"Fresenius, Donate Life America Announce Living Donor Registry." Healio, *Nephrology News & Issues*, Oct. 28, 2019. https://tinyurl.com/yx6a9mzs.

Goldenberg, Ilan. "What I Learned from Donating a Kidney to My 70-Year-Old Father." *VOX*, Mar. 6, 2019. https://tinyurl.com/wweytg2.

Morrison, Josh. "Almost All Kidney Donors Are Proud, like Me. So Why Did One Negative Story Go Viral?" *VOX*, Oct. 11, 2016. https://tinyurl.com/z8orcs6.

"New UNOS Kidney Allocation System Narrowed Racial Gaps in Transplant." *Renal and Urology News*, June 14, 2017. https://tinyurl.com/qmedpag.

Persaud, Natasha. "Racial-Ethnic Gap in Living Donor Kidney Transplantation Widens." *Renal and Urology News*, Jan. 3, 2018. https://tinyurl.com/skj5aby.

"Presumed Consent Not Answer to Solving Organ Shortage in U.S." Healthcare-in-Europe.com. June 12, 2011. https://tinyurl.com/ryu4p8v.

Profeta, Louis M. "Forget Blood Type. Soon We'll Be Able to Transplant Organs from Different Species." LinkedIn, Dec. 14, 2016. https://tinyurl.com/vjt8xw7.

"Why 99% of Austrians Donate Their Organs." *Behavioural DESIGN*, Aug. 11, 2015.

TV, Radio, and Podcasts

Jadran, Farah. "Facebook Post Leads to Life-saving Kidney Transplant for First-time Mom." LOCAL.syr.com, May 5, 2016. https://tinyurl.com/yatyfzow.

Offen, Carol, and Crais, Elizabeth. "The Outs and Ins of Organ Transplantation." Interview by Erin Welsh. *This Podcast Will Kill You*, Feb. 9, 2021. Episode 66. https://thispodcastwillkillyou.com/

Villicana, Rafael. "What Is a Preemptive Kidney Transplant?" Interview by Lori Hartwell. *KidneyTalk* (podcast radio show), March 6, 2019. RSNHope.org., Web ID 3021. https://tinyurl.com/yxrcqkdf.

Miscellaneous

CISION PR Newswire, "At White House Organ Summit Today NKF Announced New Collaboration with Johns Hopkins University and Novartis to Nationally Launch Live Donor Champion Program." News release, June 13, 2016. https://www.prnewswire.com/.

Guinness World Records, "Longest Kidney Transplant Chain." https://tinyurl.com/hezxpebn.

Job Security for Living Organ Donation Guaranteed under Family and Medical Leave Act, Aug. 28, 2018. https://tinyurl.com/sa9qmt2.

The Kidney Project: Frequently Asked Questions by Patients. The University of California at San Francisco's bioartificial kidney project, which is in preclinical trials. https://pharm.ucsf.edu/kidney/device/faq.

Medicare Benefit Policy Manual Chapter 11: End Stage Renal Disease (ESRD), Rev. 257, 03-01-19.

Medicare Coverage of Kidney Dialysis & Kidney Transplant Services (booklet). CMS Product No. 10128 Revised December 2019.

UCLA Health, "Future Consequences of Donation." https://www.uclahealth.org/transplants/kidney/.

The White House. Executive Order on Advancing American Kidney Health. Issued July 10, 2019. https://tinyurl.com/4cfczouq.

The White House. Office of the Press Secretary, FACT SHEET: "Obama Administration Announces Key Actions to Reduce the Organ Waiting List." News release, June 13, 2016. https://tinyurl.com/wwf6jwm.

Acknowledgments

LIKE MOST BOOKS, THIS ONE started with just a basic idea: to encourage living kidney donation. The book and our goals broadened and grew gradually, gaining momentum as the book took shape. It never would have made it beyond the original idea and early-enthusiasm stages were it not for the faith and efforts of many people who believed in our goals and in our ability to fulfill them. We want to express our deep gratitude to those people who especially helped spur the book's progress.

First, we are very grateful to Dr. Ken Andreoni, not only for writing our foreword, but also for offering us valuable feedback on the rest of the book. Given that he performed both Betsy's transplant and Carol's son Paul's *and* is a former president of UNOS, he was the perfect choice to write the foreword. We are thankful for his important contributions and careful reading.

Next, we want to express our sincere appreciation for the book's contributors, who took a leap of faith in agreeing to participate when the book was still little more than a gleam in our eyes. The donors and transplant recipients eloquently and honestly shared their personal experiences from all over the country: Mike Collins and his sister/recipient Wendy Withers, Monica Sheppard, Brad Dean, Danny Ranch, Joe Reichle, Linda Watson, and Jenine Lewis. They all were extremely gracious in receiving our edits and tweaking their chapters periodically as the book evolved, and were timely in getting their work to us.

The second group of contributors, the professionals who work with kidney recipients or donors, generously contributed their expertise, insights, and advice: Kathleen Fitzgerald, Sharon Williams, and Tammy Wright.

Tammy was particularly generous with her time, in writing a chapter, frequently answering our questions, *and* reviewing a recent draft of the entire manuscript. Similarly, Jenine Lewis also read sections and offered suggestions drawn from her own experience. We are indebted to all of these contributors for their faith in us and for helping us to make this book as practical, personal, and informative as we wanted it to be.

We also want to recognize the ongoing encouragement and assistance of the excellent and caring medical professionals who helped us fine-tune the clinical aspects of the book. We want to thank the dedicated providers at the University of North Carolina Kidney Center, in Chapel Hill, where our own surgical "events" took place: in addition to Dr. Andreoni, who is now based in Florida, we are grateful to Carrie Frueauf and Amy Woodard, who reviewed large sections of the manuscript and helped us keep up to date on practices that are constantly changing; and to Clara Neyhart, Jenny Hawley, Laurie McDonald, and Liz Friedman, who provided feedback on select portions of the book.

Beyond UNC, other professionals who kindly reviewed chapters at earlier stages and responded to our numerous questions include Dr. Kevin Lee, of North Carolina Nephrology; Chad Abbott, of the University of Michigan Medical Center; and Janie Money-Neeley, retired from Harris County Community Hospital in Missouri (and a living donor herself). In addition, we want to thank the staff at Duke Transplant Center, Johns Hopkins Comprehensive Transplant Center, NYU Langone Transplant Institute, Ohio State Comprehensive Transplant Center, Oregon Health and Sciences University Clinical Transplant, Sharp Memorial Hospital Kidney and Pancreas Transplant Center in San Diego, the University of California at San Francisco Kidney Transplant Center, and others, for sharing information on their programs' practices.

We are indebted, too, to the many people from donation advocacy groups who provided information, guidance, and support, and championed our advocacy efforts: Rob Hayden, Katey Cipriani, and Andrew Fullerton of the National Kidney Foundation; Deanna Kerrigan and WELD founder Diane Brockington from Donate Life/WELD; and Ned Brooks, founder of the National Kidney Donation Organization; as well as individual dedicated advocates, such as Victoria Comella and researcher Brooklynn Wynveen, who helpfully led us to other advocates.

Several publishing professionals and author friends also kindly shared their expertise, experiences, and encouragement: Julie Allred, Barbara Williams Ellertson (who also inspired our cover-design concept), Bob Sehlinger, Brenda Cortez, Erica Eisdorfer, Ann Palmer, Tamara Miller, Frank Van Riper, Jane Gabin, Tom Wolf, Barry Prizant, and David Perry. We also want to thank our copyeditor, Fred Kameny, for his judicious editing and his responsiveness and flexibility.

We are both immensely grateful to Carol's husband, Neil, who spent countless hours combing through many drafts and making significant suggestions, from high-level conceptual aspects such as the organization of chapters and content to small but valuable edits. Neil's credentials as a writer, editor, and journalist made him an ideal personal editor for our book. We have appreciated his professional guidance throughout every step of the process.

We would also like to thank other family members, friends, and colleagues who carefully read all or large chunks of the manuscript at different stages and offered insightful and helpful feedback as engaged "first readers": Carol's daughter, Nora, who, besides reading chapters, also creatively helped us explore cover design ideas; Betsy's daughter, Rachael Wagner; Cindy Thomas; Andy Richards; Marion Di Falco; Judith Sackoff; Christine Sleight; and Laura Small.

Having family members who can provide their own perspectives on crucial events was an invaluable benefit. Carol is grateful to her son, Paul, for clarifying details and permitting her to write about intimate aspects of his difficult experiences, and to her sister Marion for supporting the entire family in so many ways when they were all so fragile in the weeks after Paul's transplant. Carol thanks her whole family for their love, support, and encouragement during the writing of this book—especially Neil, who, in addition to providing professional input, endured the years of Carol's book-related emotional ups 'n' downs.

Betsy would like to thank her husband, Mike, for his support and patience during the many meetings and time spent away from the family, as well as while writing and editing sections of the book at home. This book was a huge undertaking over years, and always Mike's support was felt. Betsy also appreciates the heartfelt contribution that her daughter, Rachael, made to the book by writing about her own feelings of anger and fear as a teenager during Betsy's transplant process and by helpfully offering suggestions to readers. Sam Wagner, Betsy's son, also deserves thanks for his support and the many kindnesses he provided to Betsy. She greatly appreciates and values the love and support of her family during the writing process.

Finally, we both would like to acknowledge the thousands of other living donors, transplant recipients, and their family members who've found comfort and support from a community of caring individuals who get it, and who try to be there for one another. The Facebook support groups that cheered our efforts these past few years provided encouragement and real-world concerns and questions for us to address in this book.

Most of all, Carol would like to thank Paul and Betsy, whose kidneys may have inspired this book but whose hearts and strength inspire her every day.

About the Authors

Carol Offen is an editor/writer and donation advocate. Her varied career has included turns as a magazine editor and writer, an author, a publications manager, a research editor, and a book editor. Early in her career she wrote features for major publications, including *Esquire, Family Circle, and Vogue.*

In 2006, Carol donated her kidney to her adult son, who had developed chronic kidney disease following a strep infection. She has been passionate about raising awareness of kidney disease ever since. She has written widely about her experience and created a website and blog, kidneydonorhelp.com. As a National Kidney Foundation advocate, Carol has spoken to members of Congress and state legislators. As a UNOS Ambassador and Donate Life/WELD member, she also shares her donation story at patient workshops and community groups—and with anyone who'll listen. Carol lives in Carrboro, North Carolina, with her husband.

Elizabeth (Betsy) Crais is an educator and researcher in speech and hearing sciences at the University of North Carolina at Chapel Hill, where she has spent most of her career. She has co-authored or co-edited several books and has been published in numerous professional journals and presented at professional meetings in the United States and internationally. Her area of expertise is identifying and intervening with young children with autism spectrum disorder and other disabilities.

In 2004, Betsy, who has polycystic kidney disease, received a kidney transplant; two of her sisters also had transplants. In 2021 she had a kidney-liver transplant from a deceased donor. She has served as a transplant mentor and often speaks to prospective kidney recipients and their families in patient workshops. Betsy lives in Chapel Hill, North Carolina, with her husband.

Index